D0668516

101 AMAZING USES for GINGER

FAMILIUS

```
. . . . . . . . . . . . . . . .
:                              :
:          TO JEFF             :
:                              :
. . . . . . . . . . . . . . . .
```

Copyright © 2017 by Susan Branson
All rights reserved.

Published by Familius LLC, www.familius.com

Familius books are available at special discounts for bulk purchases, whether for sales promotions or for family or corporate use. For more information, contact Familius Sales at 559-876-2170 or email orders@familius.com.

Reproduction of this book in any manner, in whole or in part, without written permission of the publisher is prohibited.

DISCLAIMER: The material in this book is for informational purposes only. It is not intended to be a substitute for professional medical advice, diagnosis, or treatment. Always seek the advice of your physician or other qualified healthcare provider with any questions you may have regarding a medical condition or treatment. Never disregard professional medical advice or delay in seeking it because of something you have read in this book.

Library of Congress Cataloging-in-Publication Data
2017932168

Print ISBN 9781945547126
Ebook ISBN 9781945547478
Hardcover ISBN 9781945547485

Printed in the United States of America

Edited by Lindsay Sandberg
Cover design by David Miles
Book design by Brooke Jorden and David Miles

10 9 8 7 6 5 4 3 2 1

First Edition

101 AMAZING USES for GINGER

REDUCE MUSCLE PAIN, FIGHT MOTION SICKNESS, HEAL THE COMMON COLD, AND 98 MORE!

Susan Branson

CONTENTS

INTRODUCTION

WHAT IS THIS KNOBBY ROoT?

Most know ginger as a yellow spice in the baking aisle of the grocery store. It's in the same family as turmeric and cardamom, other familiar spices. Bought fresh, it has beige- to brown-colored skin covering knobby, fingerlike projections. These projections are called *rhizomes* and are the horizontal stems of the plant that are found underground and from which both the upright stem and roots of the plant grow. Underneath the skin is the wonderfully aromatic ivory- to yellow-colored flesh. When cut into, a spicy, lemony, and pungent smell fills the air.

The ginger root shows up in stores all around the world, but it is native to the warmer climates of Asia—particularly India and China—although Australia, Brazil, Jamaica, West Africa, and parts of the United States now cultivate it. It's a perennial, so it comes up every year. It has long, narrow green leaves and green-purple flowers that look somewhat like orchids.

Ginger is teeming with more than one hundred fifteen chemical constituents in the rhizome, with at least fourteen found to be bioactive. The main groups of bioactive compounds are called *gingerols* and *shogaols*, and the amount of each of these depends on where the ginger was grown, the commercial processor, and the form it is in—fresh, dried, or processed.

It is the gingerols in particular that give the ginger its pungent flavor and are thought to be responsible for most of the pharmacological actions, which is how ginger can have such a varied and significant impact on our bodies. Ginger is metabolized and readily absorbed after ingestion,[1] meaning that ginger gets broken down into its chemical components so they can be used by our bodies for a number of benefits. It is not surprising, then, to see some of its therapeutic benefits in these areas. Among its most notable actions are its anti-inflammatory, antioxidant, antiemetic (nausea), analgesic (pain), antipyretic (fever), antitussive (cough), and antibiotic properties. This book shows how ginger can be used to treat an incredible assortment of conditions from colds to cancer and how it is effectively used in natural beauty treatments.

WHERE DID IT COME FROM?

Having been coveted and cultivated for as long as five thousand years, ginger has stood the test of time. Our ancestors were onto something. Originating in the beautiful jungles of Southern Asia, the people of India and China are thought to be the first to have used ginger to treat their ailments and as a flavoring agent in their food and drinks. Chinese records indicate those who grew acres of ginger enjoyed great wealth, likely using it in trade. Even Confucius was a fan, reportedly never being without it at meals.

Ginger was then brought from India to Ancient Rome over two thousand years ago by Arab traders and used extensively by the

Romans for its medicinal properties until the Roman Empire fell. Pedanius Dioscorides, a Greek physician traveling throughout the Roman Empire, would collect local medicinal herbs and record his findings, notes which he later turned into *De Materia Medica*, a vast reference book on the medicinal properties of over a thousand herbs. He wrote that ginger "is right good with meat in sauces, or otherwise in conditures: for it is of an heating and digesting quality; it gently looseth the belly, and is profitable for the stomach, and effectually opposeth itself against all darkness of the light; answering the qualities and effects of pepper."[2] Undoubtedly, ginger was used as a digestive aid, for flavoring, and as a warming agent. The Greeks prized ginger so highly, they mixed it into their breads to create the first gingerbreads.

Unfortunately, with the fall of Rome, ginger was lost in Europe until the eleventh century. Once reintroduced, it quickly gained popularity, surpassed only by black pepper in the fourteenth century. It was so coveted that it became very expensive. One pound of ginger was the equivalent in trade to one sheep. Queen Elizabeth I of England was noted to be especially fond of preserved ginger and had it used in the making of sweets. She is credited with the invention of the gingerbread man, a cookie popular with kids today.

Toward the end of the Middle Ages and the emergence of world travel, ginger made its way to the New World with the Spanish Conquistadores. It reached the rest of the world with Western European explorers and travelers. Soon, everyone was enjoying this magnificent plant.

WHAT'S THE BEST WAY TO BUY AND STORE GINGER?

Fresh ginger is easy to find in the produce section of almost all grocery stores. Fresh ginger has the highest amounts of the active component gingerol and will impart superior flavor compared to other forms. Young ginger, or spring ginger, is harvested at five months and is not yet mature. The skin is thin and edible, the rhizomes tender, and the flavor mild. It will have pink tips and be lighter in color than mature ginger. Mature ginger is harvested a few months later and has a tougher skin that must be carefully peeled away before eating. The skin should still be smooth and firm with a light sheen. For a more pungent flavor, this is the way to go. Be careful not to buy too old, though. Fresh ginger loses moisture and becomes woody and stringy as it ages. Stay away from ginger that is wrinkled or moldy—sure indications of decay. Store your fresh ginger unpeeled in the refrigerator for up to three weeks or in the freezer for six months or longer.

Powdered ginger is the dried rhizome that has been ground. It is found in the spice aisle in the grocery store. Crystallized ginger or candied ginger is cooked in sugar syrup, air-dried, and rolled in sugar. Both powdered and crystallized ginger should be kept in a tightly sealed container in a cool, dark, dry place—like your pantry—for up to two years, although potency can begin to fade after six months.

Pickled ginger is sliced ginger preserved in sweet vinegar and appears either bright red or pink. It was once found only in Asian markets, but it is readily found in many grocery stores today. Store it in the refrigerator in its container for two to three months.

Preserved ginger comes from fresh young roots that are peeled, sliced, and cooked in a sugar-salt mixture. It can be found in Asian and specialty markets. This, too, can be stored in the pantry for up to two years.

Lastly, dried roots are exactly how they sound: whole or sliced ginger dried in the sun, oven, or dehydrator. Store them in a sealed container in the pantry for up to two years.

WHAT'S THE BEST WAY TO PREPARE AND USE GINGER?

Fresh spring ginger does not require peeling, while mature fresh ginger should be peeled using a knife or vegetable peeler. The ginger can then be sliced, grated, minced, julienned, or puréed. There are an abundant array of dishes that call for the use of ginger to add flavor and spice. Powdered or ground ginger is used in much the same way as fresh ginger, although the measurements are not equivalent. About one tablespoon of fresh ginger can be substituted for roughly one sixth of a teaspoon of ground ginger. While they can be interchangeable in recipes, fresh ginger tends to be better in savory dishes like stir-fries and soups. Ground ginger works better in baked goods like gingerbread and pumpkin pie or in spiced drinks like ginger tea and ginger ale. Ginger has been used in spiced drinks for a long time. In the nineteenth century, English pubs set out ginger for their patrons to sprinkle into their beer.

Crystallized ginger is not used as a spice in food but rather to add sweetness as well as flavor. It is commonly found in chutneys, preserves, sweets, and glazes. Preserved ginger is also sweeter and most frequently added to desserts. Pickled ginger is eaten on its own to freshen breath or as an accompaniment to sushi and sashimi to cleanse the palate in between pieces.

Ginger supplements are available on the market and are advertised as natural health products that can alleviate nausea, soothe digestion, calm anxiety, and improve sexual and cardiovascular health and emotional and physical well-being. They can be purchased online and in health food stores.

Beauty products abound with ginger as an ingredient. While it's commonly used as a fragrance in soaps and cosmetics, the real interest is in the effects ginger can have in creating lush, shiny hair, smooth, strong nails, and toned, clear skin.

HOW MUCH SHOULD I USE?

The amount of ginger that can be eaten depends on whether the person is an adult or child. Most studies on ginger have used anywhere from 120 milligrams (a pinch) up to 3 grams (1 2/3 teaspoons) a day. A general recommendation is to not consume more than 4 grams (2 1/5 teaspoons) a day. It's important to remember that everything we put in our bodies has an effect, and when it comes to using food for therapeutic purposes, the lowest effective dose is best.

Children under two years of age should not be given ginger. Kids and teenagers can have 1–2 grams (1/2–1 teaspoon) of ginger a day for nausea, stomach cramps, and headaches. The dosage depends on body weight, so get your doctor's input in figuring out the child's correct dose. Pregnant women may also want to seek the advice of their doctor before taking ginger. It is thought to be safe for the developing baby, but medical conditions and drug interactions need to be considered.

IS TAKING GINGER SAFE?

The US Food and Drug Administration considers ginger a safe food additive. Most people can tolerate doses under 5 grams (2 3/4 teaspoons) a day, but any more than that can cause stomach pain, heartburn, diarrhea, drowsiness, or sore mouth and throat. If it is put on the skin, especially if it is concentrated essential oil of ginger, it can cause a rash.

If medications are taken, ginger could possibly interfere with the way they work. Every individual is unique, so unexpected reactions may occur in anyone. Anticoagulants and antiplatelet drugs taken with excessive amounts of ginger could increase the risk of bleeding. Diabetes drugs and too much ginger could cause low blood sugar. Calcium channel blockers taken to reduce blood pressure may have an additive effect with ginger and result in blood pressure dipping too low. As always, just have a conversation with your doctor before starting a new supplement and determine if there's any possible problem with any medications you are already taking.

CHAPTER 1

FOR THE SMART FOODIE IN YOU

NUTRITIONAL BOOST: VITAMINS

Ginger is a good source of life-sustaining vitamins. Relatively small amounts of ginger are consumed compared to other foods like meats, whole grains, and vegetables. Because of this, the quantity of vitamins obtained through ginger is small but significant. Vitamins B1, B3, B6, C, E, and folate in ginger each have their own unique role in helping the body in growth, digestion, elimination, and overall vitality. With the exception of the vitamins our body creates on its own (for example, some B vitamins, vitamin K, etc.), most vitamins can be obtained only through food.

Ginger contains both water-soluble and fat-soluble vitamins. The water-soluble ones are mainly the B and C vitamins. As their names suggest, they dissolve in water. They are not stored in the body and, once ingested, have only a matter of hours to act before they are eliminated. It is very important to consume vitamins B and C on a daily basis. All the others are fat-soluble vitamins and are stored in the body's fat tissues. These vitamins can be mobilized as needed. Because there is a ready supply (assuming adequate nutritional intake), the body can go longer periods without having to obtain these from the diet. Ginger consumed as part of a nutrient-dense diet helps provide these vitamins in sufficient amounts to perform their functions as described below.

1. VITAMIN B1

Also known as thiamine, this vitamin is needed to enhance circulation, help in the formation of blood, and prevent the accumulation of fatty deposits on arterial walls. It also plays a role in the formation of the myelin sheath, which is the cover surrounding some nerves that is essential for them to fire properly. If sufficient levels of vitamin B1 are lacking, the nerves are more sensitive to inflammation.

Our digestion also suffers when we have insufficient B1. Thiamine is needed in the formation of hydrochloric acid, the substance that breaks down our food. It helps maintain proper muscle tone in the stomach and intestines. This assists in moving the food through the digestive process. Evidence shows that a deficiency of vitamin B1 can result in gastrointestinal disorders, irregular heartbeat, loss of some nervous tissue response, depression, and fatigue.

2. VITAMIN B3

This vitamin has several names but is most commonly known as *niacin*. It is involved in more than fifty metabolic reactions in the body and is essential in the breakdown of carbohydrates, fats, and proteins. Like vitamin B1, niacin is needed in the production of hydrochloric acid in the stomach. It further aids the digestive system through its involvement in the secretion of bile and stomach fluids.

Niacin also plays a role in the cardiovascular system by stimulating circulation and reducing cholesterol levels. It is very important in maintaining a healthy nervous system and normal brain function and has been used to treat neurologic problems. A deficiency of vitamin B3 can result in mental confusion, skin disorders, loss of appetite, fatigue, and oral problems including canker sores, sore tongue, and swelling of the mouth.

3. VITAMIN B6

Vitamin B6 or pyridoxine is readily absorbed from the small intestine and is involved in more bodily functions than almost any other nutrient. One of its major roles is to help maintain the body's sodium and potassium balance needed for proper electrical functioning of the heart, nerves, and musculoskeletal system. It can balance fluids, making it important for those suffering from water retention. Like the other B vitamins above, pyridoxine is needed for the production of hydrochloric acid in the stomach. However, vitamin B6 is not just important in the breakdown of food but also in the absorption of fats and protein, too. This vitamin plays a positive role in heart disease, cancer immunity, and depression. A deficiency of vitamin B6 can result in insomnia, irritability, anemia, acne, and morning sickness in pregnant women.

4. VITAMIN C

Vitamin C is often seen in cosmetic products. No wonder, as one of its most important functions is in the formation and maintenance of collagen. Collagen gives our bodies support and structure. It is a main component of skin, hair, and nails, and as we lose collagen, the signs of aging set in. Collagen supports the body's healing processes and can speed wound healing after injury or surgery.

Vitamin C also protects the body from degenerative processes through its antioxidant function. It stimulates the immune system and can help prevent and treat infections and disease. Even external influences that cause inflammation like viral, bacterial, and fungal infections can be treated with vitamin C. Not to be outdone by the other vitamins, it, too, plays a role in preventing heart disease by reducing plaque formation on arterial walls and subsequent blood clots. Symptoms of bleeding gums, slow healing of wounds, urinary tract infections, general weakness, excessive hair loss, and aching bones and joints may indicate a deficiency of vitamin C.

5. VITAMIN E

There are actually eight antioxidant compounds that make up vitamin E. As an antioxidant, this vitamin helps combat free radical damage to tissues from pollution, chemical exposure, and processed foods. The tissues most sensitive to oxidation from free radicals are the skin, liver, breasts, testes, and eyes.

Vitamin E is very important in preventing heart disease. It decreases blood clotting and raises "good" cholesterol levels. Taken internally or externally, vitamin E is commonly used to heal dry skin, repair burns or abrasions, or even fade scars. A deficiency of vitamin E could lead to heart disease, premature aging, diarrhea, irritability, or weakness.

NUTRITION

HEALTH

COSMETICS

6. FOLATES

Even though folate is a water-soluble vitamin, a nine-month supply can be stored in the liver. It is used in red blood cell production and is significant in preventing anemia. And it's not only important for red blood cells: folate is needed for the growth and reproduction of all cells. This is why it is essential for pregnant women or those trying to become pregnant to take folic acid supplements. It ensures a ready supply during fetal development when there is rapid cell multiplication. With respect to the infant's growth, folate plays a crucial role in the development of the nervous system and can prevent neural tube defects.

Just as vital is folate's role in reducing atherosclerosis, strengthening immunity, and combating depression and anxiety. Folate deficiency can result in bleeding gums, paleness, diarrhea, insomnia, irritability, and fatigue.

NUTRITIONAL BOOST: MINERALS

Minerals make up about 5 percent of our body weight, mostly in the skeleton. Ginger contains the macrominerals potassium, magnesium, phosphorus, and calcium and the microminerals iron and zinc. These are essential for the body in energy production, formation of blood and bone, regulation of muscle tone, and maintenance of healthy nerve function. Macrominerals are needed in larger quantities than microminerals, but all are equally vital for good health. They are so important that vitamins cannot carry out their jobs properly without them. The only way to get minerals is from the earth, from intake of food and water. Ginger can be consumed with a variety of other nutritious foods to ensure the body has high-enough levels of minerals to perform their functions as outlined below.

7. POTASSIUM

One of the major roles potassium plays is as part of the sodium-potassium pump in the body. This regulates the water balance and acid-base balance in the blood and tissues. The importance of this is to regulate the heartbeat and help generate muscle contractions. A direct effect of these functions is the control of blood pressure. For those with high blood pressure, increasing potassium intake rather than decreasing sodium intake is actually a more reliable way to lower it! Signs of potassium deficiency include high blood pressure, irregular heartbeat, muscle fatigue, swelling of the ankles, and constant thirst.

8. MAGNESIUM

Considered the "anti-stress" mineral, magnesium is a natural tranquilizer that relaxes the skeletal muscles and the smooth muscles of blood vessels and the gastrointestinal tract. Magnesium is

NUTRITION

important to the cardiovascular system because it can prevent heart attacks, lower blood cholesterol, and treat hypertension. Research shows magnesium also helps play a role in preventing osteoporosis and certain forms of cancer and in alleviating the symptoms of premenstrual syndrome. Experiencing muscle spasms, gallstones, irregular heartbeat, or excessive body odor may indicate a magnesium deficiency.

9. PHOSPHORUS

HEALTH

Most phosphorus is deposited in the bones, a bit in the teeth, and the rest in other cells of the body. It is involved in the formation of bones and teeth, cell growth, blood clotting, and kidney function. It's important to have enough phosphorus to help keep strong and regular contractions of the heart. Too much, however, can compete with calcium for absorption in the intestines and cause an imbalance in the ratio of phosphorus to calcium. If less calcium is available, problems with bone health can result.

Another major role of phosphorus is in the conversion of food to energy. Deficiencies can cause fatigue, bone pain, irregular breathing, numbness, trembling, and anxiety. Our North American diet often provides too much phosphorus, so deficiencies are rare.

10. CALCIUM

COSMETICS

Calcium is the most abundant mineral in our bodies. It is best known for its role in the development and maintenance of healthy teeth and bones. As people get older, particularly women, ensuring adequate levels of calcium intake is extremely important to prevent osteoporosis. It plays an important part in the cardiovascular system by helping maintain a regular heartbeat, reducing cholesterol, assisting in blood clotting, and potentially lowering blood pressure. Calcium is also known to help prevent cancer and is useful in keeping the skin looking healthy. Inadequate calcium levels can lead to osteoporosis, brittle nails, irregular heartbeat, muscle cramps, and insomnia.

11. IRON

Iron functions primarily in the formation of hemoglobin, an essential molecule that carries oxygen in red blood cells to all the tissues of the body. Without this oxygen, these tissues would not be able to survive. Similarly, iron is a key component of myoglobin, which also holds oxygen and carries it to the skeletal muscles and heart. Sufficient amounts of these molecules give the body the energy for muscle performance. Unfortunately, iron is commonly deficient in the diet. Symptoms of this can include a lack of energy, pale lower eyelids, dizziness, rapid heart rate, a craving for ice, and spoon-shaped nails.

12. ZINC

This mineral deserves lots of consideration because it performs so many wonderful functions in the body! It builds collagen to keep

NUTRITION

skin supple and smooth. Collagen deteriorates with age and tends to break down more rapidly in women than in men. Zinc is known to reduce colds and infections, speed the healing of wounds, and aid in the prevention of acne. In men, zinc is crucial in prostate gland function. The depletion of zinc in soil and from food processing has caused a deficiency of this mineral in many people. White spots on fingernails, acne, frequent infections, slow wound healing, thinning hair, red stretch marks, or a loss of sense of smell or taste may indicate low zinc levels.

NUTRITIONAL BOOST: FLAVOR NOTES

13. SPICE IT UP!

HEALTH

COSMETICS

There is just something about the cooler temperatures and longer days of fall that have many people turning to comfort food. Maybe it's to stave off the chill of impending winter or give people something to look forward to as they cozy up indoors. Whatever the reason, taking favorite traditional foods and turning up the heat on them will give a nice change of pace. Ginger has a wonderfully strong smell reminiscent of lemon and pepper and has been described as hot, tangy, zesty, and spicy. It is known as a stimulating herb and increases circulation by getting the blood flowing. Ginger warms the body from the inside out and brings about a feeling of calmness. Adding ginger to dishes can completely change the mood of a food, giving it a bit of pep. It pairs well with produce (pumpkin, carrots, cauliflower, and collard greens), herbs (basil, lemongrass, and mint), meats (seafood, chicken, and beef), and other ingredients like honey, cream, and soy sauce. Really, it's up to the imagination and—of course—the taste buds to try food pairings that are worthy of seconds.

Try mixing ginger with soy sauce and using in a beef-and-broccoli stir-fry or a salad dressing with ginger, garlic, extra virgin olive oil, and lemon. Ginger will add zest to carrot cake and spice to sweet potato and cauliflower soup. Try this ginger recipe that calls for fresh, chopped ginger.

GINGER VEGGIE STIR-FRY
ALLRECIPES.COM

1 tablespoon cornstarch
1 1/2 cloves garlic, crushed
2 teaspoons chopped fresh ginger root, divided
1/4 cup vegetable oil, divided
1 small head broccoli, cut into florets
1/2 cup snow peas
3/4 cup julienned carrots
1/2 cup halved green beans
2 tablespoons soy sauce
2 1/2 tablespoons water
1/4 cup chopped onion
1/2 tablespoon salt

1. In a large bowl, blend cornstarch, garlic, 1 teaspoon ginger root, and 2 tablespoons vegetable oil until cornstarch is dissolved. Mix in broccoli, snow peas, carrots, and green beans, tossing to lightly coat.

2. Heat remaining 2 tablespoons vegetable oil in a large skillet or wok over medium heat. Cook vegetables in oil for 2 minutes, stirring constantly to prevent burning. Stir in soy sauce and water. Mix in onion, salt, and remaining teaspoon ginger. Cook until vegetables are tender but still crisp.

14. PICKLED GINGER TO CLEANSE THE PALATE

During the holiday season when one delectable dish after another is eaten or at a wedding feast serving an extended six-course meal, it's advisable to cleanse the palate in between dishes so as to properly enjoy the sumptuous tastes of all the foods without intermingling flavors. Pickled ginger is often used as a palate cleanser and is a common accompaniment to sushi and sashimi. It is eaten between pieces to ready the senses for the next bite. The best pickled ginger comes from fresh young ginger that has been marinated in vinegar and sugar. It's the acidic vinegar that acts with the ginger to neutralize competing flavors in the mouth. The young ginger lends a tender and sweet flavor over the more mature form. It is easy to make your own pickled ginger at home.

HOMEMADE PICKLED GINGER (GARI)
ALLRECIPES.COM

8 ounces fresh young ginger root, peeled
1 1/2 teaspoons sea salt
1 cup rice vinegar
1/3 cup white sugar

1. Cut the ginger into chunks and place them into a bowl. Sprinkle with sea salt, stir to coat, and let stand for about 30 minutes. Transfer the ginger to a clean jar.
2. In a saucepan, stir together the rice vinegar and sugar until sugar has dissolved. Bring to a boil, then pour the boiling liquid over the ginger root pieces in the jar.
3. Allow the mixture to cool, then put the lid on the jar and store in the refrigerator for at least one week. You will see that the liquid will change to slightly pinkish in a few minutes. Don't be alarmed—it's the reaction of the rice vinegar that causes the change. Only quality rice vinegar can do that! (Some commercial pickled ginger has red coloring added.) Cut pieces of ginger into paper-thin slices for serving.

15. GINGER TEA FOR COLD WINTER DAYS

Being outside in cold weather can chill the bones. The neck stiffens, the upper shoulders ache, the nose runs, and a sore throat may start. A quick and effective way to rid the body of these symptoms is to drink ginger tea. Ginger tea has a warming effect that increases circulation and can induce perspiration. It's especially useful to drink during cold and flu season because it has antiviral and antibacterial properties that can help fight the dreaded symptoms and get folks back on their feet. Ginger tea can be used to settle the stomach, quell nausea, soothe anxiety, and provide pain relief.

Ginger tea had a colorful use in the early 1900s at afternoon dances. A tea of ginger, cinnamon, chamomile, and orange slices was served to the ladies in an attempt to get the blood flowing and inspire them to let loose!

You can purchase ginger tea in most grocery stores, or it can be made at home.

GINGER TEA

1 teaspoon unpeeled ginger root
Boiling water

1. Grate ginger root into a cup. Pour boiling water over it and let it steep for 2 minutes.
2. Strain or let the ginger settle to the bottom.

16. GINGER AND CHOCOLATE: AN UNUSUAL PAIRING

If there's anything more decadent than chocolate, it's chocolate and ginger. Pairing the bitter taste of the chocolate with the spicy flavor of the ginger creates an unparalleled sensory experience. For those that like a little sweetness, using crystallized ginger will satisfy that craving. Try this chocolate-and-ginger cake.

SWEET-AND-SPICY CHOCOLATE CAKE
ALLRECIPES.COM

1 1/3 cups all-purpose flour
1/3 cup unsweetened cocoa powder
1/2 teaspoon baking powder
1 cup chopped dried apricots
1 cup boiling water
5 ounces almond paste
3/4 cup white sugar
4 eggs
2/3 cup whole milk
3 ounces bittersweet chocolate, chopped
2/3 cup finely chopped crystallized ginger
3/4 cup unsalted butter, melted

1. Preheat oven to 350 degrees F (175 degrees C). Grease and flour a 9x5-inch loaf pan. Sift together flour, cocoa, and baking powder.
2. Soak chopped apricots in boiling water for 1–2 minutes. Drain and pat dry with paper towels.
3. In a large mixing bowl, mix almond paste and sugar with an electric mixer until the mixture looks sandy. Beat in eggs one at a time; beat for 2 minutes after each addition. Continue beating for about 10 minutes; the mixture should look thick and creamy.
4. Mix in milk and then the flour mixture. Mix only to combine the dry with the wet ingredients. Do not overbeat. Fold

NUTRITION

HEALTH

COSMETICS

in apricots, chocolate, crystallized ginger, and melted butter. Transfer batter to a prepared loaf pan.

5. Bake in preheated oven for about 1 hour or until done. Cool for 10 minutes in pan. Remove from pan and place on a wire rack to cool completely.

CHAPTER 2

FOR THE HEALTH ENTHUSIAST IN YOU

MANAGING DISEASE

17. ALLERGIES

They can strike in spring when pollen fills the air, at a friend's house when that cute ginger kitten rubs against a leg, or after eating the most satisfying lunch at the local popular seafood restaurant. Allergic reactions can cause minor irritations that result in a stuffy nose, watery eyes, or mild headache or potentially be so severe as to threaten life. They happen when the immune system reacts to a substance, whether it's swirling through the air, absorbed through the skin, or eaten for lunch. While these substances don't cause a problem for most people, the immune system doesn't recognize them in those with allergies. It sees them as unwelcome invaders and launches an attack against them. Specific antibodies are produced for each allergen that the body identifies as harmful. Every time a person comes in contact with that allergen, the allergic response is activated.

There is no cure for allergies, but there are many over-the-counter and prescription drugs available to help ease symptoms. Among these are antihistamines, decongestants, and corticosteroids. They can cause drowsiness, high blood pressure, insomnia, irritability, restricted urine flow, muscle weakness, fluid retention, and weight gain. And these are just some of the side effects. This seems like trading one set of symptoms for another.

For a more natural approach, try ginger. The compound 6-gingerol in ginger strongly inhibits allergic reactions. It suppresses compounds involved in the body's allergic response, thereby preventing or alleviating allergy symptoms. This was demonstrated by the oral administration of a 2 percent ginger diet in mice with induced hay fever. The severity of sneezing and nose rubbing was significantly reduced.[3] Ginger can be taken every day without any of the side effects of traditional allergy drugs, eliminating any undesirable reactions and saving the consumer money.

18. ALZHEIMER'S

Alzheimer's disease—a form of dementia—is a progressive brain disorder that is irreversible. It can begin with greater memory loss and result in wandering and getting lost, repeating questions, and some personality and behavioral changes. As it progresses, memory loss and confusion grow worse and people may have trouble recognizing friends and family, carrying out multistep tasks, or coping with new situations. In the late stage, brain tissue shrinks significantly and communication becomes difficult. Alzheimer's patients become completely dependent on others for care and often become bedridden. In most people with Alzheimer's, symptoms begin in their midsixties. Early onset may have genetic factors in play, and late onset arises from complex brain changes that occur over decades. Current treatment approaches encourage patients to focus on mental function and manage behavioral symptoms. Several medications have been approved by the FDA for the treatment of these symptoms.

In South Asia, ginger rhizome has been used for centuries to treat dementia. One study showed that 6-shogaol is the bioactive ingredient in ginger that reduces memory impairment by inhibiting glial cell activation. These are the most abundant cells in the central nervous system. They play a key role in the destruction of neurons, which are needed for memory and other cognitive functions.[4] Ginger slows down the process by which the brain loses its cells and can help keep people active, alert, and lucid for longer.

19. ANOREXIA

This psychological disorder is characterized by needless weight loss, extremely low body mass index, an irrational fear of gaining weight, and a distorted body image. The causes are complex and can stem from childhood traumas, social pressures, hormone imbalances, or nutritional deficiencies. Genetics is thought to play a part, but the role it plays is not yet fully understood. Anorexics may show an obsession with calorie counting and diets. Physical symptoms can include depression, thinning hair, the absence of menstruation, and a sensation of feeling cold. Medical and nutritional treatments as well as psychological therapy are used to overcome this disorder.

One major obstacle is stimulating the appetite. Having denied the body sufficient food for prolonged periods, the appetite wanes. Without the desire to eat or an appetite to motivate this desire, the road to recovery becomes more difficult. This is where ginger comes in. Ginger's beautifully strong aroma can stimulate the salivary glands and release digestive enzymes in the mouth. This induces a craving for the food having this mouth-watering effect. Ginger can also boost metabolism, which is needed for the body to perform all the complex processes necessary to maintain a healthy body. Anorexics don't consume enough food to allow the body to have a good metabolic rate or meet all its energy demands.

After stimulating the appetite and boosting metabolism, ginger helps the body absorb the nutrients by triggering the secretion of gastric and pancreatic enzymes. Food is broken into its component nutrients and made available to the body to help the healing process begin on a physical level. Mentally, ginger stimulates the mind and improves concentration, which may help renew interest in food and provide the willpower to follow dietary recommendations.

20. ASTHMA

Asthma is a chronic condition in which the airways leading to the lungs are inflamed. When exposed to triggers (chemicals or situations that impact the body), the airways swell and produce extra mucus. The passageway for air narrows, and breathing becomes more difficult. Symptoms include coughing, shortness of breath, wheezing, and chest pain. Anyone can develop asthma, although some are genetically predisposed to it. Triggers can be allergens, both environmental and food based, or other substances like smoke, pollution, or changes in the weather. Learning what your specific triggers are goes a long way in asthma management. Doctors often prescribe controller medications like corticosteroids and long-acting beta agonists and sometimes leukotriene modifiers to help manage the condition. Short-acting beta agonists are prescribed to quickly relieve symptoms by relaxing and opening the airways.

A common side effect of asthma medication is thrush, a yeast infection in the mouth. Ginger is a known antifungal and can combat this symptom. Chew on ginger after taking the medication or drink ginger tea. This has the added benefit of helping to remove mucus from the throat and lungs. Other side effects of asthma medications include headache, nausea, skin rash, stomach pain, and diarrhea. Read on to find out how ginger can help alleviate all these symptoms.

It is not only the symptoms but also the cause of asthma that can be controlled with ginger. A study was presented at The American Thoracic Society in 2013 that found that adding ginger to a short-acting beta agonist enhanced the opening of the airways. Other studies have confirmed the role of ginger in preventing airway constriction. A 70 percent aqueous extract of ginger inhibited airway contraction in mice lung cells[5] and significantly and rapidly relaxed human airway smooth muscle cells. Further study showed it was ginger's 6-gingerol, 8-gingerol, and 6-shogaol that caused the rapid relaxation response.[6] Ginger can provide an alternative or complementary approach to asthma management.

21. ATHEROSCLEROSIS

This is a disease in which plaque builds up inside the arteries, the blood vessels that carry oxygen-rich blood to the body. Plaque collects along the arterial walls and is made up of fat, cholesterol, calcium, and other substances. Over time, the plaque hardens and makes the arterial path smaller. If not treated, blood flow can become so constricted that a heart attack, stroke, or even death may result. Atherosclerosis is a very common disease and often exists without any outward symptoms. The risk factors include an unhealthy diet, lack of exercise, and smoking. It is not surprising, then, that the main treatment is a change in lifestyle to incorporate healthy choices.

Ginger is effective in treating patients with high blood fat levels. A double-blind study tested 3 grams a day of ginger against placebo and found triglycerides and cholesterol were significantly reduced in the patients treated with ginger.[7] Another study reported that ginger can inhibit vascular smooth muscle cell growth, which is involved in the formation of arterial plaque. Currently, this growth is stopped by drugs released from stents that have been placed in patients after bypass surgery. This surgery is performed to restore normal blood flow to an obstructed coronary artery. The 6-shogaol in ginger has been proven to perform the same function as these drugs released from stents and can perhaps be used with them in the future.[8]

22. BLOOD CLOTS, BLOoD THINNER

Blood clots are necessary to stop bleeding in an open wound, but they can also form in the body where they can be dangerous. Blood clots can form in arteries and veins in an attempt to repair tissue damage by laying down layers of fibrin and platelets. Clot formation within the arteries and veins is a problem because these clots slow the flow of blood. They can block blood vessels completely at their site of origin or they can break off and plug a vein or artery elsewhere in the body. This can be extremely serious and can lead to heart attack or stroke. Depending on where the clot is located, treatment can be with either anticoagulation medications or with acetaminophen or ibuprofen to manage pain and inflammation. However, some side effects of anticoagulants include severe bruising, bleeding gums, vomiting blood, chest pain, and prolonged nosebleeds.

Ginger is proposed as an antiplatelet treatment for patients with blood clots without the side effects of traditional anticoagulant drugs. Antiplatelet compounds decrease platelet aggregation and inhibit clot formation. A study testing gingerol compounds like those in ginger found they significantly inhibited platelet formation, and some were as effective as or more effective than aspirin.[9] Another study confirmed gingerol compounds and their derivatives' superiority to aspirin as antiplatelet agents.[10] Adding 1 gram of ginger to 10 milligrams of nifedipine (a drug used to treat high blood pressure and chest pain) in hypertensive patients may be more effective than taking either alone.[11] Ginger, then, could be used to manage heart disease by reducing damage to the blood vessels.

. . . .

23. BREAST CANCER

Breast cancer starts when cells of the breast begin to grow out of control and form a tumor. Tumors are cancerous if they grow and spread into other areas of the body. It is much more common in women, but men can get breast cancer, too. Early detection can be made through mammograms before symptoms begin. If not detected early, breast cancer can cause bloody discharge from the nipple or changes in the shape or texture of the breast or nipple. It can also be felt as a lump. Treatment may involve radiation, chemotherapy, or surgery.

An extract from ginger was tested on two breast cancer cell lines to see if it suppressed the growth of cancer cells. It did. Not only did it stop the growth of cancerous cells and colony formation, but ginger also showed selective action in not affecting the viability of normal breast cells.[12] This is promising news in the fight against breast cancer.

24. BRONCHITIS

Bronchitis is a respiratory disease characterized by the inflammation of the lining of the bronchial airways of the lungs. Acute bronchitis can result from a cold or other respiratory infection causing the mucus membranes to swell and air pathways to narrow. Chronic bronchitis is more severe and is a constant inflammation of the lining of the bronchial tubes, most often caused by smoking. People with bronchitis have coughing spells and often cough up mucus. Chest pain, fever, chills, and fatigue are other symptoms. Acute bronchitis often goes away on its own after a short time, while chronic bronchitis persists and often requires cough medicine, asthma inhalers, or antibiotics if a bacterial infection is suspected.

Studies have shown ginger to have a role in preventing airway constriction. A 70 percent aqueous extract of ginger inhibited airway contraction in mice lung cells[13] and significantly and rapidly relaxed human airway smooth muscle cells. Ginger's 6-gingerol, 8-gingerol, and 6-shogaol caused the rapid relaxation response.[14] Ginger has been used for centuries to treat the symptoms of cold and flu and is touted as a natural cure for cough. It expands the lungs and loosens phlegm. Ginger tea will ease a sore throat, break up congestion, and reduce coughing. Slice up some fresh ginger and boil in water to ensure the active ingredients are drawn into the tea.

25. COLON CANCER

Colon cancer begins with the formation of benign clumps of cells called *polyps* in the large intestine. Over time, these polyps can become cancerous. In the early stages, no symptoms are common, but as the disease progresses, patients experience changes in bowel habits, rectal bleeding, abdominal pain, fatigue, and unexplained weight loss. Like most cancers, treatment is often radiation, chemotherapy, surgery, or a combination of these.

Numerous studies on the effects of ginger in suppressing colon cancer cells have been undertaken. A randomized, blinded study on individuals taking 2 grams of ginger root supplement for 28 days showed ginger lowered the levels of inflammation in the colon and was found to be tolerable and safe.[15] This can help reduce the risk of developing colon cancer. Another study found that ginger significantly decreased the incidence of cancer and the number of tumors in rats that had induced colon cancer.[16] Ginger was also shown to inactivate colon cancer cells through DNA fragmentation[17] and decrease their growth.[18] Ginger shows promise as an effective antitumor agent to complement conventional treatments.

26. DIABETES

Diabetes is a disease that affects the way the body handles glucose, resulting in high levels of this sugar in the blood. There is type 1 diabetes, in which the pancreas produces little or no insulin, type 2 diabetes, in which the pancreas does produce insulin but the body doesn't use it as well as it should, and gestational diabetes, a form of high blood sugar affecting pregnant women. Some people are genetically predisposed to diabetes, but being overweight is also a risk factor. Feelings of thirst, frequent urination, fatigue, tingling, numbness in the hands or feet, and blurry vision are all signs of diabetes. Managing diabetes involves exercising, improving diet, and monitoring blood glucose levels. For many, daily insulin injections are needed.

The high incidence of diabetes makes finding an easy and natural alternative to manage this disease very desirable. Studies toward this end have uncovered ginger as an effective agent. In a randomized, double-blind, placebo-controlled trial, diabetes patients received either 3 grams of ginger powder or placebo a day for 8 weeks. Ginger significantly lowered fasting blood glucose levels over placebo.[19] The 6-gingerol present in ginger was tested in laboratory rats with high blood fat and insulin levels. Ginger reduced blood fat levels, body weight, blood glucose levels, and blood insulin levels.[20] These symptoms are often seen with insulin resistance in type 2 diabetes. Another study using rats showed that those who were fed ginger achieved better glucose tolerance and higher blood insulin levels than untreated rats.[21] Ginger may be valuable in controlling blood sugar levels and managing the effects of diabetes in humans.

27. GASTRIC CANCER

This is stomach cancer. The cells in the lining of the stomach begin to grow uncontrollably and can spread to nearby organs or to the lymph vessels and nodes where it can be carried to other parts of the body. It grows slowly and tends to only show symptoms in later stages. Stomach cancer is more common in men than women and in those older than their midsixties. The nitrites and nitrates in processed meats have been shown to cause stomach cancer in lab animals, so skipping the pepperoni on pizza or the bacon with eggs is a good idea. Smoking can double the risk of stomach cancer, and secondhand smoke is just as dangerous. A third common cause of stomach cancer is infection with *Helicobacter pylori* (*H. pylori*) bacteria. Most people with this infection never develop stomach cancer, but long-term infection can cause inflammation of the inner lining of the stomach, giving rise to precancerous changes. Symptoms can include nausea, vomiting, loss of appetite, a sensation of feeling full, abdominal pain, and heartburn. Conventional treatments include medications, surgery, chemotherapy, and radiation.

Enter ginger. Ginger can help alleviate the symptoms of stomach cancer and shows promise in tackling the disease itself. It can quell nausea and reduce vomiting and pain. Ginger can stimulate the appetite by inducing the secretion of salivary enzymes in the mouth with its spicy aroma. It can increase gastric motility to help reduce the "full" feeling that some experience, and it has been shown to be a natural remedy for heartburn. As for the cancer itself, 6-shogaol, a compound in ginger, was shown to reduce the viability of gastric cancer cells by damaging structures inside the cells called microtubules, effectively stopping cell division.[22] This suggests new cancer cell production is reduced, slowing the progression of disease.

28. HIGH CHOLESTEROL

Cholesterol is a waxy, fat-like substance found in cells. It is necessary for the body to make vitamin D, hormones, and bile acids that help digest food. We produce cholesterol on our own, but we also get it in saturated fat and cholesterol-laden foods. It comes in two forms: the good and the bad. High cholesterol is when there are high levels of cholesterol in the blood, both good and bad. When there is too much of the bad cholesterol in the body, however, it can build up in the arteries and increase the chances of getting coronary heart disease. Plaque containing cholesterol builds up inside the arteries and causes partial or full blockage, leading to the narrowing and hardening of the arteries. This can lead to a heart attack or stroke. Statins are drugs commonly prescribed to lower the bad blood cholesterol. Taking statins can cause intestinal problems and muscle inflammation.

Cholesterol levels respond well to changes in diet. Eating foods low in saturated fats and reducing intake of animal products, which are the primary contributors of cholesterol in the diet, will do wonders. Ginger has been studied for its effect on blood fat levels. A double-blind, controlled clinical trial has shown that patients with high levels of fat in their blood significantly reduced cholesterol and triglyceride levels by about 90 percent and 36 percent more than placebo by taking 3 grams of ginger a day over 45 days.[23] Ginger is also a source of vitamin B3, which is known to lower the bad and raise the good cholesterol in the body. Consuming ginger appears to be effective in managing cholesterol.

29. LEUKEMIA

Leukemia is a cancer of the body's blood-forming tissues. Abnormal white blood cells are produced by the bone marrow and don't function properly. They can't perform their main role of fighting infections. These cells grow and divide more rapidly and continue to live when the normal cell life cycle is over. They begin to crowd out healthy cells, and symptoms begin to develop. The exact causes are not understood, but it's thought that both genetic and environmental factors are at play. Symptoms can include fever or chills, fatigue, bone pain, frequent infections, excessive sweating at night, recurrent nosebleeds, and swollen lymph nodes. Like other cancers, chemotherapy, radiation, and medications are used to treat leukemia. Sometimes stem cell transplants are given to replace diseased bone marrow with healthy bone marrow.

Ginger boosts the immune system, which can greatly benefit leukemia patients by helping to provide protection against infections. There are several compounds in ginger that have been shown to be effective in fighting leukemia's cancer cells. Ginger's 6-gingerol causes the cancer cell's DNA to break apart and suppresses the disease's ability to transform normal cells into leukemia cells.[24] The 6-shogaol in ginger inhibits tumor growth and triggers cell death in human leukemia cells.[25] These compounds show promise as antitumor agents in leukemia.

NUTRITION

30. LIVER CANCER

This is a cancer that begins in the cells of the liver. A mutation in the DNA causes cells to grow rapidly and eventually form a tumor. It's not clear what the cause of liver cancer is in many cases, but certain chronic infections with hepatic viruses in the liver may lead to it. Symptoms appear in the later stages of the disease and include weight loss, abdominal pain, yellowed skin (jaundice), and vomiting. Surgery to remove part of the liver, liver transplant, chemotherapy, and targeted drug therapy are some treatment options.

Ginger shows promise as a complementary agent and has been proven to be effective in causing the death of liver cells through ginger's compound, 6-shogaol. The 6-shogaol activates an enzyme that is known to mediate programmed cell death. The cancer cells shrink and fragment, causing their death.[26] Ginger can also reduce nausea and vomiting, stimulate the appetite to minimize weight loss, and assist in reducing abdominal pain. It can boost the immune system to help the body fight this disease. Ginger, then, can help improve overall health and optimize liver function during this difficult time.

HEALTH

31. LIVER DAMAGE

The liver is the largest internal organ in the body. It filters toxins out of the bloodstream to prevent them from damaging tissues. When the liver tissue itself becomes damaged, it is able to regenerate and make new, healthy tissue. When the damage gets too extensive,

COSMETICS

however, liver disease sets in and the liver no longer functions as it should. A number of conditions can cause liver disease, including hepatitis A, B, and C, cirrhosis of the liver, nonalcoholic fatty liver disease, and alcoholic hepatitis. Symptoms include abdominal swelling and pain, bruising, fatigue, loss of appetite, and jaundice.

A study published using laboratory animals showed the administration of ginger and chicory significantly improved liver damage and restored the liver's blood composition to normal. This effect happened whether ginger was taken alone or in combination with chicory.[27] Ginger may also help prevent or treat nonalcoholic fatty liver disease, which is becoming more prevalent today with the rise in diabetes. It provides this protective effect by targeting the factors that contribute to this condition. It reduces oxidative stress on the liver, decreases insulin resistance, and inhibits inflammation.[28] The antioxidant ability of ginger can also guard against alcohol-induced liver damage.[29] Ginger has the potential to be used as a natural supplement for the prevention and treatment of liver disease.

32. OSTEOARTHRITIS

Osteoarthritis is the most common form of arthritis, characterized by inflammation of the joints. The joints provide the connection between bones that allow for movement. They are cushioned by cartilage to allow the joint to move smoothly and easily. In osteoarthritis, the cartilage breaks down and causes the inflammation. Extra fluid is produced in the joint, resulting in swelling. This disease affects many people as they age due to natural wear and tear. Heredity plays a role, as does injury from trauma or disease. Those afflicted suffer from joints that are painful, creaky, stiff, and swollen.

Their range of motion is reduced, particularly in the hands, feet, spine, hips, and knees. Reducing the stress on the joint cartilage is recommended to alleviate some of the symptoms. This involves losing weight and avoiding certain activities. The goal of treatment is to reduce pain and inflammation to allow for more comfortable movement. Medications are taken as pills, creams, gels, and even injections into the arthritic joint. Side effects of these can include gastrointestinal distress such as stomach upset, diarrhea, or ulcers.

Ginger is touted as having anti-inflammatory and pain-relieving properties that can reduce swelling and alleviate pain, the two common symptoms of osteoarthritis. Clinical research has shown that patients with osteoarthritis of the knee that took a 250 milligram ginger extract four times a day for three months had significantly reduced pain compared to placebo.[30] This effect was noted after three months of treatment with ginger, indicating that it must be taken daily for at least that period to have an effect. A different extract from a combination of ginger and a related plant commonly known as Siamese ginger was tested in osteoarthritis patients. After six weeks of taking two doses of 255 milligrams a day, stiffness and pain upon standing and after walking was significantly reduced.[31] Ginger has even been compared to ibuprofen. A 500 milligram dose of ginger extract taken twice daily in one group of patients with osteoarthritis of the hip or knee was tested against a 400 milligram dose of ibuprofen taken three times a day over a one-month period. Both significantly reduced pain and swelling. Ginger was found to be just as effective as ibuprofen.[32] Ginger, then, can be used to manage osteoarthritic symptoms. If patients choose to go with conventional medical treatments, ginger can help alleviate the gastrointestinal side effects these medications often cause.

33. OSTEOPOROSIS

Osteoporosis is a bone disease in which the body can't produce enough new bone to replace old bone removal. The process of bone absorption and replacement happens continuously in the body, and in those with osteoporosis, bone mass decreases over time. A decrease in mass and density results in weakened bones that are more likely to break. It is more common in women than men because women have lower bone masses. Osteoporosis is known as a silent disease because it doesn't produce symptoms and diagnosis is often made after a bone has been broken. This disease runs in families, so if a parent or grandparent had osteoporosis, there is an increased chance the next generation will have it too. Certain diseases and medications can also increase the likelihood of developing osteoporosis. A healthy diet sufficient in bone-producing minerals, weight-bearing exercises, and medication are recommended for management and treatment.

Ginger contains a compound called *zerumbone*. Zerumbone was tested in mice to see if it could prevent human breast cancer–induced bone loss. It was discovered that it could decrease the destruction and disappearance of bone tissue in a dose-dependent manner.[33] This suggests a potential role for ginger as a therapeutic agent in osteoporosis.

34. OVARIAN CANCER

Ovarian cancer is the uncontrolled growth of cells in the female reproductive organs called the ovaries. It often goes undetected in the early stages. This cancer easily spreads to the surrounding areas of the bladder, bowel, and abdomen before traveling to other sites in the body. The exact cause of ovarian cancer is unknown, but evidence strongly supports a genetic link. Symptoms are often nonspecific but can include bloating, pelvic pain, loss of appetite, and urinary problems. Surgery and chemotherapy are generally used to treat ovarian cancer.

Research at the University of Michigan Comprehensive Cancer Center found that ginger can destroy ovarian cancer cells. Ginger was able to induce cell death through cell self-destruction and through digestion by lysosomes, organelles in most cells that contains digestive enzymes that can degrade and destroy cellular components. They found that ginger induced ovarian cell death at a similar or better rate than some chemotherapy drugs typically used for treatment. In cultured ovarian cancer cells, other research showed that it is the 6-shogaol compound in ginger that causes significant cancer cell inhibition. Ginger may have potential in the prevention and treatment of ovarian cancer.[34]

35. PANCREATIC CANCER

Pancreatic cancer begins in the tissues of the pancreas, the organ that lies horizontally behind the lower part of the stomach. The pancreas secretes enzymes to aid in digestion and hormones to regulate the metabolism of sugars. Cancer develops when cells mutate and grow rapidly and continuously. They live long after normal pancreatic cells have died and eventually form into tumors. This disease often goes undetected and spreads rapidly. Symptoms begin to appear later in its progression and may include loss of appetite, weight loss, blood clots, depression, upper abdominal pain, and jaundice. Treatment options are surgery, chemotherapy, and radiation.

Two compounds in ginger have been tested and show potential as new therapeutic candidates in controlling pancreatic cancer. Ginger's 6-gingerol suppressed the growth of human pancreatic cancer cell lines by stopping cancerous cells from dividing and by inducing cell self-destruction.[35] And zerumbone, another ginger compound, induced cell death in several pancreatic cancer cells.[36] Because current drug candidates to suppress pancreatic cancer are lacking, these compounds from ginger may be considered.

36. PARKINSON'S

Parkinson's is a progressive disorder of the central nervous system that can cause tremors, stiffness, slow movement, and loss of balance. Nerve cells become damaged in the brain, causing dopamine levels to drop. This leads to abnormal brain activity that manifests itself in these characteristic symptoms. The cause of Parkinson's disease is largely unknown, but it is believed that genetic predisposition combined with environmental triggers plays a role. As this disease progresses, cognitive function declines, and those afflicted

NUTRITION

can experience insomnia, depression, constipation, fatigue, or bladder problems. Parkinson's can't be cured, but medications can be taken to improve the symptoms. The medications increase or substitute for dopamine in the brain. Some advanced cases may opt for surgery to implant electrodes in a specific part of the brain to help reduce the symptoms. Exercise, physical therapy, and speech language therapy are often recommended.

Free radicals have been implicated in the development of Parkinson's disease. These are uncharged molecules that are highly reactive and set off a chain reaction in a cell, which can destroy it. Antioxidants neutralize free radicals and protect the cell from damage. *Zingerone*, a compound extracted from ginger root, was tested in the brains of mice for its antioxidant ability. Oxygen-scavenging activity was increased, decreasing the presence of damaging free radicals in the mouse brains. Its direct antioxidant activity as well as its ability to increase an enzyme that neutralizes free radicals provides the basis of ginger's neuroprotective effects. This indicates that zingerone in ginger may be a possible treatment for Parkinson's disease.[37]

HEALTH

37. PROSTATE CANCER

This is cancer that occurs in a man's prostate, the small gland that produces seminal fluid to nourish and transport sperm. It can begin when some cells in the prostate mutate and begin to grow and divide rapidly. They live long after normal prostate cells and come together to form tumors. These tumors can grow to invade nearby tissue, or some abnormal cells can break off and spread to other

COSMETICS

parts of the body. Some prostate cancers grow slowly and remain confined to the prostate. These often require minimal treatment and monitoring. Other types can be more aggressive and spread quickly. These need the more invasive treatments, which usually consist of surgery, chemotherapy, radiation, or hormone therapy. Advanced cases may cause difficulty urinating, slow urine stream, blood in the semen, erectile dysfunction, and bone or pelvic pain.

Using a dietary agent like ginger to manage prostate cancer is easily accessible and cost-effective. The results of several studies suggest its use may prove beneficial. Whole ginger extract was fed to mice daily at 100 milligrams/kilogram of body weight for eight weeks. Prostate tumor size shrunk by 56 percent, while normal, healthy cells were not affected.[38] Ginger extract was also used to test its effectiveness on an aggressive prostate cancer cell line. It was found to significantly inhibit the cancerous cells from forming colonies.[39] Ginger demonstrates effectiveness in managing prostate cancer.

38. RENAL FAILURE

Renal failure, or kidney failure, is a condition in which the kidneys lose their ability to remove waste products from the blood and balance fluids. Acute cases of renal failure occur when the kidneys suddenly lose their filtering ability and dangerous levels of waste products build up in the blood. This happens over a short period of time and requires intensive treatment. Complete recovery from acute renal failure is possible. Conversely, chronic renal failure is progressive and irreversible. Symptoms are due to the buildup of waste products in the body and include weakness, shortness of breath, fatigue, and confusion. Abnormal heart rhythms and sudden death can follow. Prevention is the best course of action and involves controlling blood pressure and diabetes. If the disease has progressed too far, dialysis or transplants are needed.

Ginger has antioxidants that scavenge free radicals in tissues. A study that fed rats a 5 percent diet of ginger found that ginger was able to reduce renal injury and protect the kidneys by removing the free radicals that cause (in part) the injury.[40] A similar study tested the effects of ginger on chronic and acute kidney failure. The kidneys were protected by ginger's antioxidant activities as well as its anti-inflammatory activities. Ginger can be considered for a role in slowing the disease progression and may delay the need for dialysis.[41]

39. RHEUMATOID ARTHRITIS

Rheumatoid arthritis is an autoimmune disorder in which the immune system mistakenly attacks its own body tissues. The lining of the joints become painfully swollen and can lead to bone erosion and joint deformity over time. Symptoms can spread to other non-joint tissues of the body. It's not known what causes this disease, but genetics combined with environmental triggers are suspected. This chronic disease is without a cure and is managed mostly through medications. Nonsteroidal anti-inflammatory drugs, steroids, or disease-modifying antirheumatic drugs can be prescribed to reduce pain, swelling, and joint damage. Possible side effects include digestive problems, liver and kidney damage, heart problems, thinning of bones, diabetes, weight gain, and severe lung infections.

NUTRITION

HEALTH

COSMETICS

Fortunately, ginger has been proven to be effective in reducing inflammation and pain associated with rheumatoid arthritis without any of the side effects. Powdered ginger was used as a dietary supplement by fifty-six patients suffering from rheumatoid arthritis, osteoarthritis, or general muscular discomfort over a period ranging from three months to two and a half years. More than three quarters of those with arthritis experienced some degree of relief in pain and swelling, and all those with muscular pain reported relief. One of the ways ginger works is by preventing the production of prostaglandin and leukotrienes, compounds involved in inflammation.[42] Severity of swelling in the joints should be reduced and the associated pain lessened.

40. SEPSIS

Sepsis is a serious and potentially life-threatening complication of an infection. The immune system activates macrophages—white blood cells that digest cellular debris and foreign substances—to fight the infection, but this response can trigger inflammation throughout the body. A series of changes can take place that damages multiple organs and may lead to their failure. If the condition progresses, septic shock sets in and blood pressure drops dramatically. Death can result. Early treatment with antibiotics and intravenous fluids can reverse the condition. Sometimes vasopressors are used to bring up blood pressure. Any type of infection, whether it is bacterial, viral, or fungal, can cause sepsis.

Macrophages produce powerful chemicals that promote systemic inflammation, as seen in sepsis. Macrophages exposed to

6-gingerol from ginger in several doses inhibited the production of these inflammation-producing chemicals without interfering with the macrophage's ability to capture foreign bodies for destruction.[43] The 6-gingerol's anti-inflammatory ability can be used to reduce inflammation in conditions like sepsis and still allow the body to fight the infection.

41. SKIN CANCER

This common form of cancer is the abnormal growth of skin cells resulting from a mutation that allows the cells to grow out of control and form a cancerous mass. It develops most often on the sun-exposed areas of the skin, but it can develop in areas protected from the harmful ultraviolet (UV) radiation of the sun that often causes it. Other factors, such as exposure to toxic chemicals or a weakened immune system, may also be responsible. There are three types. Basil cell carcinoma appears most often on the face and neck and can look like a waxy bump or scar-like lesion. Squamous cell carcinoma is most frequent in areas of the skin exposed to the sun and can look like a red nodule or a flat lesion with a scaly, crusted surface. Melanomas can appear anywhere and are characterized by large brownish spots with darker speckles or dark lesions on the hands, feet, or mucous membranes. Moles that change in color or size, that bleed, or that have irregular borders may be melanoma. Surgery, radiation, or topical medications are the conventional treatments for skin cancer.

Ginger shows promise as an agent to protect against skin cancer. Cancerous human skin cells in a study were treated with 6-gingerol from the rhizome of the ginger plant. Ginger's 6-gingerol was able to inhibit the growth of the cancerous skin cells by triggering a series of reactions that activated cell death. This suggests 6-gingerol can be used in the treatment of skin cancer.[44] Results of a similar study show that topical application of ginger's 6-paradol or 6-dehydroparadol compounds decreased the number of mice exhibiting tumor growth and the number of tumors on each mouse.[45] This adds further evidence of ginger's effectiveness as a potential treatment for skin cancer.

42. ULCERATIVE COLITIS

Ulcerative colitis is an inflammatory bowel disease that causes long-lasting inflammation in the innermost lining of the large intestine. The symptoms can vary depending on where the inflammation is located in the large intestine and are usually mild to moderate with periods of remission. Some signs of ulcerative colitis are diarrhea with blood or pus, rectal bleeding, abdominal or rectal pain, an urgency or inability to defecate, fever, fatigue, and weight loss. Treatment options include anti-inflammatory drugs or immunosuppressants. Severe cases may need surgery to remove the colon and rectum.

Ginger has potential to be used in the management of chronic inflammatory conditions like ulcerative colitis. A study in male rats showed ginger to be effective in alleviating the symptoms of ulcerative colitis when consumed over ten days. The improved condition of the disease is attributed to ginger's anti-inflammatory and antioxidant properties. At its highest dose, it was even found to be as effective as sulfasalazine, a commonly prescribed anti-inflammatory drug for ulcerative colitis.[46] This research supports the use of ginger as a valuable agent in the treatment of inflammation in this intestinal disease.

43. ULCERS

Ulcers are holes in the protective lining of the stomach, small intestine, and esophagus. Sores develop that may cause stomach pain, bloating, heartburn, nausea, and fatty food intolerance. Infection with *H. pylori* is thought to be the main cause. Overuse of painkillers, smoking, stress, and heavy alcohol use are other contributing factors. If *H. pylori* are present, treatment involves a course of antibiotics to kill the bacteria. Medications to neutralize, block, or reduce the production of stomach acid are often prescribed. It is imperative that the use of painkillers, smoking, and alcohol is greatly reduced or stopped.

Over a period of two years, the gastro-protective effects of an aqueous extract of ginger was evaluated in laboratory rats and compared to the effects of omeprazole, a medication prescribed for stomach ulcers. The ginger root extract inhibited gastric ulcers by nearly 58 percent when administered at 400 milligrams/kilogram of body weight. Its gastro-protective effect was comparable to omeprazole and has shown itself to be a promising anti-ulcer agent.[47] Another study in laboratory rats clearly demonstrates that extracts of ginger can protect the stomach and intestinal lining from ulcers. Ginger also inhibits gastric acid secretion and the growth of *H. pylori*.[48]

MANAGING SYMPTOMS

44. COLD AND FLU

Common colds and seasonal flu are respiratory illnesses caused by different viruses. They are highly contagious, and a person can become infected by touching a surface such as a doorknob, stair railing, or bathroom faucet. If the virus gets on the hands and the person then touches his or her mouth or nose, the virus nestles into the mucosal lining there. Breathing in air near someone who is coughing or sneezing because they are sick with a cold or the flu is another surefire way of getting the virus into the system. There are many different viruses that cause colds and flus. Unless the body has fought the exact virus before, it won't have the right antibodies ready to fight it when it enters the body. The immune system begins an attack against the new virus, and the dreaded symptoms set in. A sore throat, runny or stuffy nose, sneezing, and cough are the hallmarks of a cold. If these symptoms are accompanied by a fever, fatigue, and muscle aches, it is more likely to be the flu. There is no shortage of over-the-counter cold and flu medications, and they are available for every possible symptom. Take a walk down the pharmacy aisle to see antihistamines, decongestants, nasal sprays, cough suppressants, and throat lozenges.

An inexpensive and effective home remedy to combat these symptoms and have you feeling better sooner is to use ginger. It has been used as a natural treatment for colds and flu in Asia for thousands of years. The University of Maryland Medical Center states that cold and flu symptoms in adults can be treated by steeping two tablespoons of freshly shredded or chopped ginger root in hot water two to three times a day. Ginger is a known antiviral and can help the body get rid of the virus. It provides support to the immune system and will shorten the duration of the illness. Ginger can also reduce the symptoms caused by the virus. It helps the body perspire to cleanse toxins out of the system and brings down body temperature resulting from fever. Its pain-relieving properties can soothe sore, achy muscles, and its anti-inflammatory properties can relieve stuffy noses and congested chests. It is a natural cough suppressant[49] and can reduce the airborne spread of the virus to loved ones. This in combination with its sedative property allows for a restful night's sleep to reduce fatigue and give the body time and energy to conquer the virus.

45. COLIC

Colic is a condition in healthy babies in which they cry excessively for more than three hours a day, three days a week, for three weeks or longer. Colic is common and usually starts a few weeks after birth and continues for several months. Colic can cause babies to cry intensely for no apparent reason at predictable times of the day.

They can be inconsolable and clench their fists, scrunch up their legs, and tense their abdominal muscles. This suggests gastrointestinal discomfort and pain. It is unclear why some babies develop colic and others don't, but food allergies, underdeveloped digestive systems, and colon spasms are suspected. Gas relief medications and probiotics are sometimes used to treat colic, with variable results.

Ginger speeds up the movement of food through the stomach by increasing contractions to empty it into the small intestines.[50] It provides relief from gas and bloating by accelerating the release of gas out of the digestive tract. If intestinal spasms are bothering the baby, ginger can take care of that, too. It has the ability to relax muscle spasms and provide much-needed relief (to baby *and* caregivers!). Babies should not be given ginger directly. Instead, nursing mothers can drink ginger tea several times a day and pass on the benefits while breastfeeding.

46. CONSTIPATION

Constipation is infrequent bowel movements or difficulty in passing stools. It is very common and can be occasional or chronic. Occasional constipation is short term, while chronic constipation is having less than three bowel movements a week for at least three months. When stools move too slowly through the digestive tract, they become hard and dry. They are difficult to pass, and a feeling of not being able to empty the rectum is reported. Increasing fiber intake, fluids, and exercise are known to help increase gastric motility. If that doesn't work, laxatives and other medications that draw water into the intestines are suggested. Side effects of these drugs include bloating, gas, diarrhea, nausea, vomiting, and rectal pain.

Ginger root has long been used for gastrointestinal support. It has been shown to enhance the transport of charcoal meal through the intestinal system of mice fed both whole ginger extracts and isolated compounds from the root.[51] This effect was confirmed by another study that showed an increase in the rate of gastric emptying in rats when ginger was taken one hour before eating.[52] This is significant for those suffering from constipation and who want a natural way to stimulate their system to move food through the body for elimination.

47. COUGH

Coughing is the body's reaction to irritated airways or a reflex action to remove mucus and foreign material from the lungs and upper airways. Smoke, dust, allergies, asthma, some medicines, bronchospasms, or an inhaled object causes dry coughs. Wet coughs result when mucus drains down the back of the throat from the sinuses or comes up the airways from the lungs. Infections, viruses, lung disease, postnasal drip, and smoking can cause mucus-inducing wet coughs. People commonly buy expectorant medications to break up congestion and suppressants to try to stop the cough. These medications can become addictive and cause dizziness, drowsiness, nausea, and vomiting, even at recommended dosages.

Ginger has been used to manage coughs for thousands of years. A recent study extracted polysaccharides (long-chain carbohydrates) from ginger rhizomes and orally administered them to

NUTRITION

HEALTH

COSMETICS

guinea pigs. Coughing was significantly inhibited, and no signs of addiction were noted.[53] Ginger is also known to break down and remove mucus in the airways, relieving some coughs. The University of Maryland Medical Center suggests adding a drop of ginger oil or a few slices of ginger to a steaming bowl of water. Lean over the bowl and inhale deeply and slowly, being careful not to burn the nasal passages. Drinking ginger tea several times a day provides the benefits of ginger, too. Combining freshly grated ginger, fresh lemon juice, and raw honey is a wonderfully refreshing and soothing tea to ease coughing and its accompanying sore throat and congestion.

48. DECONGESTANT

A cold, upper respiratory tract infection, asthma, or allergies can all cause nasal or chest congestion. Nasal congestion is also known as a stuffy nose and can be accompanied by sinus pain. The membranes in the nose become irritated and inflamed and produce mucus. Little, if any, room is left for air to pass. Chest congestion is when membranes in the airways of the chest and lungs become swollen and irritated. They also overproduce mucus in an attempt to rid the body of the irritant causing the reaction. It's uncomfortable, annoying, and takes its toll on our overall feeling of well-being. No wonder many of us turn to over-the-counter decongestants for help. Decongestants work by either shrinking swollen blood vessels to open up the airways or by thinning and loosening the mucus caught in the lungs, airways, and nose to make it easier to cough or blow it out.

Ginger is becoming more commonly recognized for its natural decongestant and antihistamine properties and is being incorporated in herbal remedies for kids and adults. It has a warming effect that can loosen and thin mucus and an anti-inflammatory effect that relieves swollen airways. Gingerol is one of ginger's compounds known to suppress mucus production and reduce inflammation. One of the best ways to use ginger in this instance is in ginger tea. Adding fluids helps thin the mucus, as does the heat and steam from the tea. Try cutting some fresh ginger slices and boiling them in water. Add some warmed coconut milk and a teaspoon of local raw honey for a ginger-coconut tea latte.

49. DEPRESSION

Depression is a mood disorder that causes a deep sadness and a loss of interest in activities. It affects how a person feels, thinks, and behaves and can cause not just emotional problems but physical problems as well. Clinical depression may occur once in a person's lifetime or reoccur multiple times. This feeling of sadness and loss can cause insomnia, loss of appetite, poor concentration, fatigue, suicidal thoughts, and physical symptoms like backaches and headaches. Changes in the body's hormone levels may cause or trigger depression. Modifications in the way brain chemicals work and the effect that has on maintaining stable moods is thought to play a major role in depression. Psychological counseling and antidepressant medications are often prescribed. Antidepressants can cause a wide range of side effects, including nausea, insomnia, blurred vision, weight gain, fatigue, and sexual dysfunction.

Ginger is known to play a role in mental health. Several of its compounds have been found to positively affect mood. Gerianiol is found in the essential oil of ginger. Mice exposed to chronic mild stress were treated for three weeks with gerianiol, and it was found to alleviate depression-related behaviors. This antidepressant-like effect may prove useful in the treatment of clinical depression.[54] Another test, in mice, using dehydrozingerone found in ginger rhizomes indicates that this compound has potent antidepressant effects involving important brain chemicals that act as hormones and neurotransmitters.[55] Ginger is also very safe and nonaddictive. It is an incredible alternative to the often-overused antidepressants.

50. DIARRHEA

Diarrhea describes loose, watery stools. It is very common and usually lasts a few days, although prolonged diarrhea can indicate a medical condition like irritable bowel syndrome. Stomach cramps and pain, bloating, fever, nausea, and vomiting often accompany diarrhea. It occurs when the stool moves too quickly through the colon so that the colon doesn't have time to absorb enough liquid from it. The main culprits that cause diarrhea are viruses, bacteria, and parasites. Food intolerance and many medications can also cause diarrhea in susceptible people. If diarrhea persists for more than a few days, doctors may prescribe antibiotics if the cause is bacterial or parasitic.

Ginger has the power to destroy germs in the intestinal system responsible for causing diarrhea. Gingerol has antibiotic properties and has been used to treat intestinal infections and bacterial dysentery. It is said to be effective in food poisoning by eliminating abdominal pain, soothing the intestinal muscles, and reducing cramps. It stimulates intestinal enzyme activity to break down food and allow for nutrient and water absorption from it. Peristaltic movements of the bowel are slowed, and bowel movements return to normal. Ginger's reported anti-influenza compounds will attack viral infections, putting an end to the virus and alleviating diarrhea.[56] Parasitic infections by giardiasis are common in humans worldwide. Infected mice treated with ginger for seven days post infection saw reduced giardiasis viability and intestinal mucosal damage. Ginger can be used as an effective and natural alternative to relieve diarrhea with little to no side effects.[57]

51. FEVER

Fever is a temporary increase in the body's temperature. It is not an illness but a sign that something unusual is happening in the body. Mild fevers should be left untreated to allow the immune system to take care of the cause. Higher fevers are of more concern and require some intervention. Sweating, chills, fatigue, muscle weakness, and headache may accompany fevers. They are generally caused by viruses, bacteria, some medications, sunburn, inflammatory conditions, and malignant tumors. Over-the-counter medications such as aspirin, acetaminophen, or prescribed antibacterial drugs are effective in reducing fever but come with risks. Antibiotics destroy good intestinal bacteria, causing digestive upset; overuse of acetaminophen can cause kidney and liver damage; and aspirin can cause stomach pain, unusual bleeding, and weakness.

Ginger stimulates the body to produce heat, bringing body temperature up and inducing fever. This promotes sweating to remove toxins from the body more rapidly. Ginger contains vitamin C to stimulate the immune system to attack the root of the illness and find relief. It also contains zinc, known to reduce infections and, in turn, reduce the symptoms of infections like fevers. A study on the intravenous and oral administration of 6-gingerol and 6-shogaol from ginger confirms the fever-reducing activity of ginger.[58]

52. FOOD POISONING

Food poisoning is an illness caused by eating food contaminated with viruses, bacteria, parasites, or the toxins they produce. Nausea, vomiting, and diarrhea can start as soon as a few hours after eating contaminated food, or it may take up to several weeks for symptoms to show. Most cases are mild and resolve themselves within a few hours to several days. Replacing lost fluids is very important to prevent dehydration. If the cause is found to be a bacterial source, a doctor may prescribe antibiotics.

Food poisoning takes its toll and leaves the body feeling extremely fatigued and the person listless. Rest is required, but it's hard to rest when dashing to the bathroom every fifteen minutes to expel fluids. This is where ginger comes in. Ginger has proven to be effective in reducing nausea and vomiting so the body can find periods of rest and keep fluids down long enough to be absorbed. This will go a long way toward recovery. After consumption, ginger concentrates in the stomach and intestines and helps prevent abnormally strong and rapid intestinal contractions that happen with diarrhea. This reduces painful cramping and retains fluid, allowing the person to rest easier. Finally, ginger's antibacterial, antiviral, and antiparasitic properties can effectively fight the source of the food contamination to rid the body of the illness.

53. GAS

Gas can accumulate in the digestive tract. It gets there from swallowing little bits of air with our food, drink, or saliva and from the digestion of food. As gas builds up, the body needs to get rid of it, either by belching or flatulating. Everyone produces gas, and it is usually not serious. Excessive gas buildup can cause bloating, stomach cramps, and intestinal pain. To avoid excessive gas and the symptoms that come with it, a change in lifestyle and diet are usually all that are needed. Eating smaller meals more frequently, chewing thoroughly, exercising, and avoiding gas-producing foods and chewing gum are recommended.

Still, sometimes, a little outside help is needed. A randomized double-blind clinical trial on healthy volunteers studied the effects on gastric function of 1200 milligrams of ginger taken one hour before eating. Ginger stimulated muscle contractions of the stomach and increased the rate at which food was emptied.[59] This is important because food that is left too long in the stomach can ferment, causing gas. It also moves gas that has already been produced through the digestive system for expulsion. This will reduce the symptoms of pain and bloating.

54. GINGIVITIS

Gingiva is the part of the gum around the base of the teeth that becomes diseased and causes gingivitis. The gums tend to bleed easily, become puffy, and turn from pink to red. They begin to recede, and tooth decay sets in. Gingivitis is caused when hardened plaque, called *tartar*, forms below and above the gum line. Tartar is full of bacteria, and it is the bacteria that begin the infection. Plaque is formed daily on the teeth, but it can easily be removed through daily brushing and flossing. If it is left to harden into tartar, it is much harder to eliminate. This disease is common and symptoms are often mild, so most people don't know they have it. Professional teeth cleaning is needed, followed by a good oral hygiene routine at home.

An effective preventative for gingivitis is to use ginger in a mouthwash. Sixty patients were enrolled in a randomized, placebo-controlled double-blind trial. Mouthwash containing ginger, rosemary, and marigold were compared to a placebo mouthwash and an antiseptic antibacterial mouthwash known for killing bacteria and preventing their growth on tissue. The mouthwashes were used twice a day for thirty seconds. After two weeks, the ginger mouthwash was found to be very effective in the treatment of gingivitis and showed significant results over placebo. Its results were even as good as the antiseptic antibacterial mouthwash, and no side effects were reported.[60] Ginger's antibacterial properties have been demonstrated, and its use would be a safe and inexpensive addition to an oral hygiene routine for the prevention and treatment of gingivitis.

55. HEADACHES AND MIGRAINES

A headache is a pain in any part of the head and may be sharp, dull, or throbbing. It can last from under an hour to several days. Migraines are severe headaches that cause intense pain, usually on one side of the head, and are accompanied by nausea, vomiting, and sensitivity to light and sound. Migraines can come with warning signs such as blind spots in the field of vision, flashes of light, or tingling sensations on the face, arms, or legs. Migraines can be so severe that the person can't function normally and often requires rest and isolation to recover. Causes of migraines are different for everyone. Some triggers could be changes in hormone levels, food allergies, stress, some medications, sensory stimuli, or changes in the environment, like a fall in barometric pressure from an approaching storm. Regular headaches can be caused by a multitude of factors, from dehydration to too little sleep to infections. They may also be symptoms of disease. Pain-relieving medications are commonly used to deal with the symptoms. In the case of migraines, antinausea medications are also prescribed.

Ginger contains potent anti-inflammatory substances and can provide headache and migraine relief by inhibiting prostaglandins that cause inflammation and subsequent pain from compressed nerves. Several double-blind clinical trials have been conducted on the efficacy of ginger's painkilling potential. Powdered ginger and sumatriptan, a commonly prescribed drug to treat migraines and cluster headaches, were compared in one hundred patients with

NUTRITION

HEALTH

COSMETICS

acute migraines. After two hours, headache severity significantly decreased in both groups. Ginger powder was just as effective as sumatriptan—and safer.[61] Some possible side effects of sumatriptan are loss of vision, chest pain, anxiety, numbness, and stomach pain. Another study treated sixty patients for 208 migraines over a one-month period with either a combination of ginger and feverfew or a placebo. The duration and intensity of migraines decreased significantly in the ginger/feverfew group over placebo.[62] Next time a headache appears, try applying a diluted paste of ginger directly on the forehead for pain relief.

GINGER HEADACHE PASTE

1/2 cup fresh, peeled ginger
1 tablespoon olive oil

1. Add ginger and olive oil to a food processor and purée. Store in the refrigerator in an airtight container.
2. Apply directly to the forehead for headache relief.

56. HEARTBURN

Heartburn is also known as acid reflux. It occurs when acid splashes up into the esophagus from the stomach and causes a burning pain in the chest. Those who suffer from heartburn will notice that it is often worse after eating and at night. The acid travels more easily up the esophagus when bending over or lying down. Over-the-counter medications are taken to reduce or neutralize the stomach acid. These can cause nausea, constipation, diarrhea, headache, and abdominal pain. Some of these seem worse than the heartburn itself.

Ginger is an alternative treatment without these side effects and is widely used as a natural remedy for the treatment of heartburn. Its effectiveness was proven in a study that compared ginger with conventional acid-reducing drugs. Both were able to inhibit the protein responsible for gastric acid secretion, but ginger was an incredible six to eight times more potent.[63] This news will have everyone reaching for ginger the next time they have heartburn!

57. HYPOTHERMIA

Hypothermia is a life-threatening condition in which the body loses heat faster than it can produce it. They body temperature drops from a normal temperature of 98.6 degrees Fahrenheit to below 95 degrees Fahrenheit. Below this temperature, the organs cannot work properly, and if not promptly treated, hypothermia will result in heart failure and death. It's most often caused by exposure to cold and can begin with shivering, fatigue, and a lack of coordination. If conditions persist, there is a progression to slurred speech, weak pulse, and eventual loss of consciousness. Once hypothermia sets in, the only way to reverse it is to bring the body temperature back up. The best approach to treating hypothermia is to prevent it.

To that end, ginger boosts metabolism and improves the burning of stored fat in a reaction that releases heat into the body. It also has the ability to dilate the blood vessels, bringing warmer blood and heat to the skin. Individuals should include ginger in their diet to help elevate body temperature if they are often exposed to cold conditions. Most obviously at risk are those going outside

NUTRITION

HEALTH

COSMETICS

into cold weather. This especially applies to children. Their smaller bodies lose heat faster than adults, and they often ignore any warning signs if they're having fun. Inside temperatures, however, can cause hypothermia, too. Elderly adults sitting in an underheated room are in danger of losing too much body heat. As we age, the body often cannot regulate internal temperature well, and the ability to sense cold is lost. Hypothermia may set in without anyone knowing. Drinking warm ginger tea several times a day during the colder months would be of great benefit.

58. INDIGESTION

Indigestion is a term used to describe a feeling of fullness during a meal or an uncomfortable fullness after eating. It is often associated with pain, bloating, and burning in the stomach area. Eating too much, eating too quickly, eating certain types of food, or taking some medications can cause it. Smoking and anxiety also play a role. Sometimes, indigestion happens without any apparent reason. What causes indigestion in one person may not cause it in another. Each person needs to learn their triggers and avoid them. Even taking those measures is not enough sometimes, and medications are prescribed to find relief. Antacids, acid reducers, antibiotics, and antistressors can alleviate the symptoms but can also produce nausea, constipation, diarrhea, headache, abdominal pain, dizziness, weight gain, and other digestive troubles.

Ginger has been used as an effective and natural treatment for indigestion for many years and across many cultures. Studies have been performed that prove its efficacy. Ginger can decrease the burning sensation often associated with indigestion by increasing the level of prostaglandins in the stomach, which protect the lining from injury and inhibit acid secretion.[64] It can also significantly reduce indigestion-related stomach pain from ulcers. In one study, 6-gingerol in ginger inhibited gastric lesions in rats by 55 percent.[65] Ginger improves bloating by increasing the rate at which food is emptied from the stomach and intestines.[66, 67, 68, 69] The physical removal of food and gas from the stomach eases indigestion at a much quicker rate. Drinking ginger tea or eating ginger root powder one hour before a meal should allow enough time to prevent indigestion. Adding a few drops of ginger oil to carrier oil and massaging it onto the abdomen can also help relieve gas and bloating.

59. INFLAMED TESTICLES

Testicles are the male sex organs that make sperm and the hormone testosterone. Viral or bacterial infections can set in, either in the blood, from other areas of the body, or from infection in the tube that carries the semen out of the testicle. The result is tenderness, swelling, redness, pain, fever, nausea, vomiting, and blood in the semen. Most cases are treated with antibiotics to destroy the bacteria causing the infection, but this treatment is ineffective if the cause is viral.

Ginger is a strong remedy to get rid of these infections effectively. It contains both antibacterial and antiviral properties that destroy the source of the infection and anti-inflammatory properties to bring down the swelling. Because the testicles are very sensitive, even minor injury can cause a significant amount of pain. Ginger is effective here, too. It can reduce primary pain in the testicles and referred pain in the groin and abdomen. Ginger

NUTRITION

HEALTH

COSMETICS

oil diffused in carrier oil can be applied directly to the testicles to reduce pain and inflammation.

60. IRRITABLE BOWEL SYNDROME

Irritable bowel syndrome (IBS) is a common intestinal disorder of the colon. It occurs when the muscles in the intestines contract more strongly or for longer periods of time than normal or when the contractions are weak, slowing the progression of food through the body. Abnormalities in the nervous system in the colon may also be responsible. IBS doesn't cause changes in the bowel tissue, however, and does not increase the risk of cancer like the inflammatory bowel diseases Crohn's and ulcerative colitis. It does, however, affect quality of life because the onset of symptoms can be unpredictable and come at inconvenient times, causing stress for the sufferer. Abdominal pain and cramps are often the first signs that the bowel is acting up. Diarrhea or constipation commonly follows with the expulsion of excessive gas and, sometimes, mucus in the stool. It is not uncommon to experience alternating episodes of diarrhea and constipation. IBS is chronic and cannot be cured, but symptoms often go away for periods of time, affording the person some relief. It is not known what causes irritable bowel, but each person has their own set of triggers that can cause symptoms to appear. Common triggers are particular foods, stress, hormones, and other gastrointestinal illnesses. Because the cause of IBS is unknown, changes in lifestyle are recommended to manage the condition. Learning to avoid any food triggers, decreasing stress, and taking probiotics are recommended. Doctor-prescribed medicines like antispasmodics, antidepressants, and antibiotics can treat IBS symptoms but may cause other gastrointestinal upsets, weight gain, fatigue, blurred vision, headaches, and more.

Ginger has been used for centuries to treat gastrointestinal upsets. This is an easy way to get relief from IBS symptoms without having to take expensive pills. A randomized clinical study tested an herbal mixture containing ginger and two other herbs against mebeverine, a commonly prescribed drug for IBS. After eight weeks of treatment, the herbal mixture with ginger was found to be as effective as mebeverine in reducing symptoms. No adverse effects were reported.[70] Ginger takes care of intestinal cramps by soothing intestinal muscles and reducing the severity of muscle spasms. It also lessens intestinal swelling[71] and relieves pain to help ease discomfort. It speeds up the movement of food through the stomach by increasing muscle contractions that empty it into the small intestines.[72, 73] This is important because food that is left too long in the stomach can ferment, causing gas. So ginger not only reduces the opportunity for gas production but also moves any gas already present through the digestive system for quicker expulsion. Thus the painful, bloated feeling is relieved.

61. MASTITIS

Mastitis is a painful infection of the breast tissue that most often occurs in mothers that are breastfeeding their babies, although it has been known to occur in women who are not nursing. Mastitis tends to happen within the first three months of breastfeeding and usually in only one breast. If milk is not completely emptied from the milk ducts during feeding, the milk can block the duct, causing the milk to stagnate and become an inviting place for bacteria to breed. Bacteria from the mother's skin or the baby's mouth can also enter the milk ducts and cause an infection. The signs of mastitis can set in pretty quickly and cause pain, swelling, tenderness, warmth, redness, and fever. Because this is a bacterial infection, a course of antibiotics is prescribed. Over-the-counter pain relievers are often used in conjunction with the antibiotics.

The Kry people are a small ethnic group in Southeast Asia who have a long tradition of using medicinal plants for postpartum recovery. Unlike other ethnic groups living in the region, Kry women breastfeed their babies immediately after birth just like many women in our North American culture. It is not surprising, then, that Kry mothers sometimes suffer from mastitis. They don't have access to the antibiotics and pain relievers we do, but they've come up with an effective way to overcome this infection. The leaves of ginger are made into a poultice and applied to the breasts to improve milk flow and reduce pain and inflammation.[74] This lends support to studies that have demonstrated ginger's anti-inflammatory and analgesic properties, which can reduce swelling and alleviate pain. In fact, ginger should be considered as an alternative to anti-inflammatory drugs, as it has been proven to be as effective as ibuprofen in reducing swelling.[75] Ginger also has antibacterial properties to fight the infection itself and provides a way to get rid of the bacteria in the breast while keeping the good bacteria in the gut that we need for a healthy digestive tract. Antibiotics destroy the helpful bacteria in the gut, and it can take some time for the body to recover.

62. MENSTRUAL PAIN, PRIMARY

Women of childbearing years often experience pain and cramping just before or during the first few days of menstruation. Pain can be mild to severe and is described as a dull, throbbing ache in the lower abdomen, hips, back, and thighs. It usually lasts twelve to seventy-two hours and, for some, can prevent normal activities for several days. It happens when the muscles of the woman's uterus contract too strongly and put pressure on nearby blood vessels. Oxygen moving to muscle tissue of the uterus is temporarily cut off, and pain results. Over-the-counter pain relievers and hormonal birth control are used to relieve pain. Primary menstrual cramps usually occur each menstrual cycle and can be associated with other symptoms like nausea, vomiting, diarrhea, and fatigue. They are differentiated from secondary menstrual pain, which has an underlying cause like a reproductive disorder or infection.

The main objective in managing this condition is reducing pain and treating the symptoms of nausea, vomiting, and diarrhea. With these symptoms under control, fatigue should resolve itself. Ginger has often been used to relieve pain. Clinical trials specifically looking at primary menstrual pain have shown that 1000 milligrams of ginger rhizome powder taken for three days at the onset of menses relieved pain and was just as effective as ibuprofen and mefenamic acid, a nonsteroidal anti-inflammatory drug used to treat menstrual pain.[76] Another study suggested that taking 1500 milligrams of ginger root powder beginning two days before the onset of menses and continuing for an additional three days was more effective in reducing pain than starting ginger treatment at the beginning of menses. Both protocols, however, were significantly more effective at relieving pain over placebo.[77]

Ginger can also treat menstrual diarrhea. It soothes the intestinal muscles and reduces intestinal cramps by stimulating intestinal enzyme activity to break down food and allow for nutrient and water absorption. This hardens the stools. Peristaltic movements of the bowel are slowed, and bowel movements return to normal. Women prone to nausea during menses will also find that ginger reduces this symptom, too. Dosages consistent to manage pain are effective in quelling nausea.

63. MORNING SICKNESS FROM PREGNANCY

"Morning sickness" refers to nausea and vomiting in pregnancy and is most likely caused by hormonal changes in the body. It is most common in the first trimester, but it can linger throughout the pregnancy and afflict women not just in the morning but throughout the day. Most cases of morning sickness do not need treatment, but if it is really bothering the expectant mother, her doctor may prescribe vitamin B6 shots, antihistamines, or anti-nausea drugs.

Women are often told to drink ginger ale to settle the stomach and reduce nausea. This would be good advice if ginger ale actually contained any ginger. Most brands don't, instead using ginger flavoring agents. These won't impart any of the benefits of real ginger.

Instead, ginger tea made from boiling freshly cut ginger will give the antinausea benefits. Luckily for moms, ginger has been extensively studied in pregnant women and has been found to be highly effective and safe. One trial showed 500 milligrams (1/4 teaspoon) of powdered ginger extract significantly reduced nausea and, to a lesser extent, retching. No impact on birth weight, gestational age, or frequency of congenital abnormalities was found.[78] Another study showed that 1000 milligrams (1/2 teaspoon) of ginger a day significantly reduced nausea and vomiting in pregnant women[79] and was even as effective as dimenhydrinate (Dramamine) for nausea—but without the side effects.[80] Despite its proven safety, it is always advisable to check with your doctor before taking any medications during pregnancy, and ginger is no exception.

64. MOTION SICKNESS

Motion sickness is something most everyone has experienced at some point in their lives. Amusement park rides no longer hold appeal, as the up-and-down, side-to-side, circular, and jerky movements can cause severe dizziness, cold sweats, nausea, and vomiting. This illness can happen during any type of motion, including travel by air, boat, car, or train. It happens when the signals received from the eyes, the body, and the inner ear send conflicting messages to the brain. Medications are often prescribed in pill or patch form but can cause drowsiness, dry mouth, blurred vision, and disorientation.

Ginger is commonly prescribed for motion sickness and has been found to be even more effective than Dramamine to quell nausea.[81] One trial with eighty sailors prone to motion sickness showed that those who took 1000 milligrams (1/2 teaspoon) of powdered ginger had less vomiting and fewer cold sweats compared to sailors taking a placebo. Reduced symptoms of nausea and vertigo were also reported, although not statistically significant.[82] Another study treated subjects with either 1000 or 2000 milligrams (1/2–1 teaspoon) of ginger before inducing illusions of movement through various stimuli, resulting in nausea. Participants had significant reduction in their nausea, in the electrical activity in their stomachs, and in the hormone that evokes nausea.[83] This study demonstrates how ginger works in the body to counteract motion sickness. Ginger can be used before travel to prevent motion sickness or as a treatment for nausea if already queasy.

65. MUSCLE ACHES

After months of inactivity, going out for a competitive game of flag football or a vigorous evening run with a friend may seem like a good idea. However, trying to move about the next day when every muscle is stiff and sore will squelch that belief. Taking preventative measures to guard against injury-induced muscle pain or aches from overuse are something to think about for next time. Muscle aches can also result from tension, stress, or disease. The pain can be anywhere in the body and last from several hours to months. If exercise induced, muscle pain results from microscopic tears in the muscle fibers, while if disease related, it can be caused by inflammation.

Ginger has proven effective in treating muscle pain. In one study, consuming 2000 milligrams (1 teaspoon) of ginger for eleven days before exercise-induced muscle pain resulted in moderate to large reductions in the severity of pain experienced by study volunteers.[84] This decrease in muscle pain may be due to ginger's ability to reduce pain and inflammation and stimulate circulation for quicker muscle fiber repair. If you forget to take ginger as a preventative, mix two to three drops of essential ginger oil in carrier oil and massage into the achy muscle to bring quick relief. The ginger oil is absorbed through the skin where the active components can start working. Massaging can increase circulation and send the pain-relieving compounds throughout the body where they are needed.

66. NAUSEA FROM CHEMOTHERAPY

Chemotherapy is a type of cancer treatment that uses one or a combination of drugs to kill fast-growing cancer cells. The therapy commonly causes nausea and vomiting in patients, depending on which drugs are received, dosages, and whether chemotherapy is used in conjunction with other therapies such as radiation. Stress and anxiety can increase the risk of nausea that, once started, is difficult to control. This adds to the patient's fatigue and is why doctors prescribe antinausea medications to prevent nausea before it starts. There are a wide range of drugs available that are highly effective. Chemotherapy can now be done on an outpatient basis, allowing patients to continue going about their lives during treatment. While different drugs cause different side effects, common ones are diarrhea, constipation, headache, stomach and muscle pain, mouth sores, and changes in cognitive thinking.

NUTRITION

HEALTH

COSMETICS

Cancer patients undergoing chemotherapy often have anxiety about the outcome and are left feeling physically and emotionally drained. Nausea is so prevalent in this treatment and can occur even when antinausea drugs are given. Preventing it beforehand goes a long way in improving the patient's quality of life during this time. Ginger is known to reduce both nausea and vomiting and can be a useful preventative for patients. It comes with little to no side effects, but it is advisable to check with a doctor to make sure there are no known possible interactions with other medications being taken. Studies have confirmed the role of ginger in chemotherapy patients when used in addition to antinausea drugs. A double-blind, multicenter trial tested three doses of ginger against placebo in patients also taking an antinausea drug. Ginger supplementation began three days before chemotherapy treatment and continued for a total of six days. All doses of ginger significantly reduced nausea on day one of chemotherapy with 500 milligrams and 1000 milligrams (1/4–1/2 teaspoon) of ginger being most effective.[85] This data is supported by another double-blind trial resulting in ginger root powder capsules being effective in reducing nausea in both children and adult chemotherapy patients who were also treated with ondansetron and dexamethasone, two drugs administered to reduce nausea.[86] Ginger can be used alongside conventional antinausea medication administered by the patient's doctor to further reduce nausea and make the patient more comfortable.

Ginger also has gastroprotective effects and can ease diarrhea and constipation by soothing the muscles of the intestinal walls, reducing cramping, and enhancing the transport of food through the intestinal system. Ginger contains potent anti-inflammatory substances and can provide headache and migraine relief by inhibiting prostaglandins that cause inflammation and subsequent pain in blood vessels of the head. It is also known to increase concentration, a reduction of which is another potential side effect of chemotherapy.

67. NAUSEA FROM HIV/ AIDS TREATMENT

AIDS is caused by HIV, the human immunodeficiency virus, which weakens a person's immune system and their ability to fight infections. Unprotected sex and sharing needles are the most common ways of transferring the virus from an infected person to another. There is no cure for the virus, but treatment with antiretroviral therapy can slow the progression of the disease and help prevent secondary infections. While there are a number of treatment choices, almost all HIV drugs cause nausea and vomiting. It can be difficult to stay on a treatment that is miserable, even if only for a few weeks.

Ginger has been shown to reduce nausea and vomiting from motion sickness, pregnancy, and chemotherapy. Now, research has proven ginger's antinausea effectiveness in retroviral treatments administered to HIV patients. In the study, 500 milligrams (1/4 teaspoon) of ginger was taken twice a day thirty minutes before a dose of antiretroviral regimen in a study of HIV-infected patients. Both nausea and vomiting were reduced over the fourteen-day treatment.[87] Ginger supplementation lessens the discomfort of nausea from antiretroviral treatment, which likely encourages patients to continue with their therapy.

68. NAUSEA AFTER SURGERY

Postoperative nausea can happen twenty-four to forty-eight hours after surgery and can be accompanied by retching and vomiting. It's usually caused by the administration of anesthesia to the patient. This is necessary to provide temporary pain relief, muscle relaxation, and unconsciousness. Not only does nausea cause extreme discomfort, but it can also increase hospital stay time and result in the readmission of some patients. Nearly all people have had the misfortune of being nauseated at some point in their lives and know how greatly it affects their ability to maintain a normal daily routine.

In one study, taking 1000 milligrams (1/2 teaspoon) of ginger preoperatively reduced nausea and vomiting episodes in patients after gynecological surgery without any reported side effects.[88, 89] These benefits occured in a variety of surgeries in which researchers studied the postoperative antinausea potential of ginger.[90] Ginger doesn't have to be taken orally to have an effect on nausea. An anesthesia practitioner studied whether 5 percent ginger oil applied on the skin before surgery would improve postoperative nausea and vomiting. It was found that 80 percent of patients using the topical application of ginger experienced no nausea compared to 50 percent of patients who did not receive ginger oil. Both groups were also treated with conventional therapies.[91] There is no doubt that taking ginger before surgery can help with nausea from anesthesia. This can get the patient on the road to recovery much faster and enhance the overall surgical experience.

69. RADIATION EXPOSURE

Radiation is energy in particle or wave form that can cause gene mutations from long-term exposure and increase the risk of cancer. Large doses over a short period of time cause radiation sickness and lead to nausea, hair loss, organ failure, or even death. Outside, there is constant exposure to radiation from the UV rays of the sun. Indoors, medical procedures using X-rays and tomography scans emit doses of radiation. In the home, some of the culprits are microwaves, wireless internet connections, and mobile phones. Living in the modern world, it is impossible to avoid radiation exposure while interacting in society. The best thing to do to minimize the effects of exposure is to take preventative measures, whether it be from the UVA and UVB rays of the sun or from surrounding electronics.

Ginger can provide that protection. Extracts of ginger rhizome given to mice for five days prior to radiation exposure contributed to a reduction in radiation sickness and mortality.[92] Ginger provides its protection from one of its potent aromatic compounds, 6-gingerol. Pretreatment with 6-gingerol protected against UVB radiation in laboratory experiments by reducing the formation of reactive oxygen species generated by radiation exposure.[93] These molecules begin a chain reaction in the cell that ultimately destroys it. Ginger keeps the cells from significant damage and reduces the risk of developing cancer from this source.

70. SLOW METABOLISM

Chemical reactions in the body convert everything consumed into nutrients used to maintain good health and proper functioning of cells in the entire body. Some of these reactions break down compounds to be used as energy. Other reactions build compounds that the cells use to carry out their jobs and to grow and repair tissues. Many of the vitamins and minerals in ginger play a crucial role in boosting metabolism. They act as enzymes to speed up reactions in the body that are necessary to produce energy for the body's functions. Without these enzymes, the reactions would be slow or stop altogether, causing a sluggish metabolism, which impacts health.

There are many reasons for a slow metabolism. With age, muscle mass declines and fat accounts for more body weight. Muscle burns more energy than fat. Women generally have higher percentages of fat in their bodies than men, so metabolism tends to be slower in women. People on diets may restrict their calories too much, causing a slowing down in metabolism to conserve energy. Some conditions like an underactive thyroid or diabetes are associated with slow metabolisms, while certain medications and genetics play a role as well.

Ginger is a metabolism-boosting substance that can increase the burning of fat to produce heat, a process called *thermogenesis*. Eating foods that encourage the body to produce heat can rev up metabolism by as much as 5 percent and fat-burning potential by as much as 16 percent.[94] Men consuming 2000 milligrams (1 teaspoon) of powdered ginger at breakfast showed enhanced thermogenesis and reported feeling less hungry after three hours compared to men who did not consume any ginger with break-fast.[95] The 6-gingerol compound was shown to be the most potent thermogenic agent in ginger.[96] Eating spicy foods, then, can speed up a slow metabolism and help the body burn fuel.

71. SORE THROAT

A sore throat is pain, irritation, and itchiness of the throat that worsens upon swallowing. The glands of the neck might be swollen, the voice may be hoarse, and small, white patches can appear on the tonsils. The main culprits are viral and bacterial infections, but smoke, dry air, and allergies can cause a sore throat, too. When the tissues lining the throat become irritated or infected, blood rushes to the area and brings with it germ-fighting cells. The blood vessels in the tissues swell, putting pressure on the nerve endings and causing pain. Sore throats from viral infections usually last five to seven days and are treated with over-the-counter pain relievers. Bacterial infections, like strep throat, require antibiotics.

Ginger can be used to treat the symptoms and the cause of a sore throat. Ginger can lower levels of prostaglandins and leukotrienes in the body that cause inflammation and subsequent pain in blood vessels. This will make swallowing much less painful. Coughing with a sore throat can be excruciating. Ginger has been used to manage coughs for thousands of years. A recent study extracted polysaccharides from ginger rhizomes and orally administered them to guinea pigs in doses of 25 milligrams/kilogram and 50 milligrams/kilogram of body weight. Both doses significantly inhibited coughing, and no signs of addiction were noted.[97] Ginger is also a strong remedy to rid the body of infections and can effectively attack both bacterial and viral sources. Taking ginger will decrease the duration of infection and aid the immune system in destroying the germs. In the case of some bacterial infections requiring antibiotics, ginger may be supplemented alongside them to provide extra bacteria-fighting power.

72. STIMuLATION OF BREAST MILK

Nursing mothers often worry about how much milk their babies are getting. Intake can't be measured as it can in formula-fed infants. As long as the baby is gaining enough weight and has an adequate number of wet and dirty diapers, the mother's milk supply is likely fine. If this is not happening, however, support is needed. Seeing a doctor is extremely vital because the cause may not be related to milk supply.

The Kry, a small ethnic group in Southeast Asia (mentioned previously), use ginger to stimulate milk production immediately after giving birth. Instead of the root, ginger leaves are used and are made into a drink or used in a poultice and applied directly to the skin.[98] This knowledge of ginger's use has endured for many years because of its effectiveness. It is thought that ginger aids in breast milk letdown and in increasing the flow and rate of milk production.

73. SWIMMER'S EAR

Water that remains in the ear after swimming can cause an infection inside the outer ear canal. The warm, moist environment is the perfect breeding ground for bacteria that are commonly found in water. They will readily invade the skin and multiply. The infection causes itching and redness that can escalate to severe pain in and around the ear, discharge of pus, fever, and partial or complete blockage of the ear canal. To stop the infection, doctors commonly prescribe antibiotics and eardrops that contain both antibiotics and steroids. Taking over-the-counter pain medications such as ibuprofen is also recommended.

Ginger can help with all the symptoms of swimmer's ear and can even destroy the bacteria that caused the infection. It contains potent anti-inflammatory substances that can reduce swelling and redness by inhibiting prostaglandins that cause inflammation. This will allow the tissues to relieve pressure on the nerves and remove any pain. Ginger has even been found to be as effective as ibuprofen in relieving pain.[99] It also contains antibacterial agents that destroy the source of the infection so the ear tissues can regain their health.

SWIMMER'S EAR REMEDY

1 teaspoon fresh ginger
2 tablespoons olive oil

1.   Chop fresh ginger and place in olive oil.
2.   Heat gently on the stove in a double boiler for twenty minutes.

The oils from the ginger will infuse the olive oil with its active ingredients.

3. Remove the ginger from the oil. Lie on one side so that the infected ear is facing up. Using a dropper, squeeze two or three drops into the ear. Remain lying down for several minutes. Have a tissue nearby to catch any oil that leaks out of the ear after returning to an upright position.

74. TOOTHACHE

Pain in or around a tooth that is sharp or throbbing is a tooth-ache. The pain may be constant or only present when pressure is applied to the tooth and is generally a result of the tooth's nerve root becoming irritated. Swelling around the tooth and headaches sometimes occur. Some causes are tooth decay, damaged fillings, infected gums, trauma to the tooth, or teeth grinding. Dental treatment is often necessary to fix a damaged tooth. Over-the-counter pain medications are used to temporarily dull pain and inflammation.

An alternative to these medications, like ibuprofen or acetamin-ophen, is ginger. Ginger can be used to experience immediate pain relief without the side effects. It contains potent anti-inflammatory substances and can provide relief by inhibiting prostaglandins that cause inflammation, which compress the nerve of the tooth and cause pain. It has even been shown to be as effective as ibupro-fen in this regard.[100] Several double-blind clinical trials have been conducted that also support ginger as a painkiller.[101, 102] A sore, throbbing tooth may quickly find relief from ginger's powerful properties. In fact, it's been used as a home remedy for toothaches for generations. Fresh ginger can be rubbed on the gums or made into a tea to be used as a mouth rinse.

75. WEIGHT LOSS

When the body accumulates too much body fat, it increases the risk of health problems like diabetes, heart disease, and certain cancers. Losing weight can improve or prevent any weight-induced conditions. Fat accumulates on the body when more calories are eaten than burned. The body stores these excess calories as fat. Exercising and eating a healthy diet with appropriate calorie intake will help burn the stored fat and reduce body weight.

A relatively effortless way to increase the body's fat-burning potential is to eat ginger. Ginger is a thermogenic food, meaning it burns calories in the food just eaten and converts them into heat. Eating foods that encourage the body to produce heat can increase metabolism by as much as 5 percent and fat-burning potential by as much as 16 percent.[103] Men consuming 2000 milligrams (1 teaspoon) of powdered ginger at breakfast showed enhanced thermogenesis and reported feeling less hungry after three hours compared to men who did not consume any ginger with breakfast.[104] Feeling full for longer prevents snacking and the consumption of additional calories. In this way, ginger can play a role in weight management.

During the weight-loss process, people often report reaching plateaus where they no longer seem to be able to continue losing weight despite continued efforts with exercise and dieting. This is because metabolism slows down as weight is lost. Ginger can counteract this decrease in metabolism. The gingerols and shogaols in ginger activate a compound that increases adrenaline secretion.[105] Adrenaline increases the circulation of blood in the body and the intake of oxygen in the lungs. The extra oxygen is pumped throughout the body and raises energy levels by burning glucose. Just like burning fat, burning glucose consumes calories and can help the body lose weight. Ginger can amp up metabolism, which allows the body to efficiently burn calories by breaking down fat, carbohydrates, and protein and converting food into energy.

MANAGING WELL-BEING

76. CONCENTRATION

Concentration is the ability to keep the mind focused on an activity for a desired period of time. It seems that some people are able to concentrate on a task for several hours, while for others, attention begins to wane after only a few minutes. Some medical conditions interfere with the ability to concentrate, as do psychological and cognitive problems. Poor concentration may be a symptom of something else, so seeing a trained professional is important if an underlying reason for an inability to concentrate is suspected. For many, however, concentration can seem to slip as they get older and they find themselves getting bored and distracted or slipping away into daydreams. A growing body of science points to two regions in the frontal lobes of the brain that gradually shift into a seesaw imbalance with age and, with it, a decreased ability to concentrate on the task at hand. This shift begins in middle age and becomes more pronounced in older adults.[106] A study in middle-aged women showed that receiving 400 milligrams or 800 milligrams (1/5 or 2/5 teaspoon) of ginger a day over two months improved cognitive function over placebo.[107] Ginger is effective because of its antioxidants, which stop free radicals in the brain from oxidizing other molecules. This prevents the premature aging, damage, and impaired function of cells. Ginger is especially important in maintaining tissue integrity in the brain because the brain uses up to 25 percent of the oxygen in our body and runs a greater risk of oxidative damage.

77. ENERGY

Everyone has lulls of energy in their day that have them longing for a quick catnap on the couch, but instead, they often reach for caffeinated beverages to boost their energy and awaken their minds. A combination of factors can lead to low energy, and common ones are lack of sleep, poor diet, stress, and depression. Taking care to manage the source that drains energy would be a good first step to give bodies what they need to function properly and provide enough energy to happily get through the day. Going to bed earlier, cutting back on saturated fats and sugar, finding outlets to deal with stress, or talking to a therapist are all ways to do this. However, to add even more pep in your steps, try taking a little ginger every day.

Ginger can amp up metabolism to allow the body to efficiently burn calories by breaking down fat, carbohydrates, and protein and convert food into energy. The gingerols and shogaols in ginger activate a compound that raises adrenaline secretion.[108] Adrenaline increases the circulation of blood in the body and the intake of oxygen in the lungs. The extra oxygen is pumped throughout the body and raises energy levels by burning glucose.

Ginger is a thermogenic food, meaning it burns calories in the food just eaten and converts them into heat. Eating foods that encourage the body to produce heat can increase metabolism by as much as 5 percent.[109] As noted above, an increase in metabolism supplies more energy to the body. Also, stimulating the body to produce heat encourages sweating, which removes toxins from the body. Toxins are harmful and can divert the body's energy to deal with them, causing fatigue. Men consuming 2000 milligrams (1 teaspoon) of powdered ginger at breakfast showed enhanced thermogenesis and reported feeling less hungry after three hours compared to men who did not consume any ginger with breakfast.[110] Ginger sustained energy for longer without having to replenish fuel as quickly.

If depression is causing fatigue, ginger can help here, too. Geraniol found in the essential oil of ginger has an antidepressant-like effect.[111] Another compound in ginger, dehydrozingerone, has potent antidepressant effects involving important brain chemicals that act as hormones and neurotransmitters.[112] Ginger is also very safe and nonaddictive. It is an incredible alternative to the often-overused antidepressants. A simple way to energize with ginger is to apply a few drops of ginger oil on a cotton ball and inhale every so often.

78. NUTRIENT ABSORPTION

Eating a diet rich in lean protein, complex carbohydrates, good fats, and vitamins and minerals is recommended for optimal health. If the body doesn't do a good job of absorbing these nutrients, your efforts in maintaining a healthy diet may be sabotaged. It is vital that the body receive nutrients to provide the fuel to function properly. Different amounts of each nutrient are required, and some are more easily absorbed than others. If there are digestive issues, nutrient absorption may be suboptimal and overall health will be compromised.

Ginger root has long been used for gastrointestinal support. After consumption, ginger concentrates in the stomach and intestines where it exerts many effects. Ginger stimulates muscle contractions of the stomach,[113] enhances transport of food through the intestinal system,[114] and increases the rate of gastric emptying when taken one hour before eating.[115] In the intestines, ginger stimulates enzyme activity to break down food and allow for nutrient and water absorption from it.

The B vitamins in ginger are used in the formation of hydrochloric acid, the substance that breaks down food in our stomachs. With age, hydrochloric acid levels decrease and food isn't digested completely. If food is not broken down into its component parts, it is too large to pass through the intestinal walls into the blood to be carried to the cells for use. Instead, it gets eliminated with all the nutrients still in it. B vitamins are essential in the breakdown of carbohydrates, fats, and proteins so that they are able to pass through the intestinal wall. Ginger provides support to both the physical and chemical digestive processes and increases the absorption of nutrients so they are available to the body.

79. STRENGTH

How much weight a person can lift, push, pull, or throw is determined by muscular strength. Many people strength train to build muscle mass and become stronger. Lifting weights or resistance training using body weight can do this. Weight training breaks down muscles, and during repair, there is new and larger growth of muscle tissue. It is theorized that the muscles grow larger to protect the body from future stresses.

Microscopic tears in the muscle fibers can cause inflammation and pain. Ginger has proven effective in treating muscle pain. Individuals consuming 2000 milligrams (1 teaspoon) of ginger for eleven days before exercise-induced muscle pain saw moderate to large reductions in the severity of their pain.[116] This is due, at least in part, to ginger's ability to reduce prostaglandins and leukotrienes, which are associated with pain and inflammation. This shortens recovery time so that the strength training program can resume without much delay.

It appears that ginger supplementation can boost the effects of strength training, too. This was shown in a study where one group of men received 1000 milligrams (1/2 teaspoon) of ginger a day and did strength training exercises while another group of men did the same strength training exercises without supplementation. At the end of ten weeks, it was found that both groups increased their muscle mass and decreased their fat mass. The group that supplemented with ginger, however, had the most beneficial results.[117] Ginger can improve physical strength by minimizing muscle pain and inflammation during the training process and by helping to boost the effects of training.

80. TOXIN REMOVAL

There are a whole host of toxins that can invade the body. They are poisonous substances that promote infection and disease by damaging the body's cells and disrupting tissue function. Toxins can be ingested with food, absorbed through the skin, or inhaled in the air. If the toxins that invade the body are pathogens, ginger can be used to stop their spread through the body. Ginger is a known antiviral, antibacterial, and antifungal agent and can help rid the body of these toxins by preventing them from attaching to cells and causing infection. Ginger also helps the body perspire to cleanse toxins out of the system more rapidly. It does this through increasing fat burning to produce heat, a process called *thermogenesis*. The compound 6-gingerol is the compound in ginger found to be a potent thermogenic agent.[118] The immune system is the body's defense against toxins. And the vitamin C in ginger stimulates the immune system, making it even more active in seeking out and destroying toxins that have invaded the body.

NUTRITION

HEALTH

COSMETICS

81. VOCAL PERFORMANCE

Singers need to keep their voices in top condition so they can perform night after night and keep their audiences coming back. Public speakers also know the importance of protecting their voices if they want to convey their messages or knowledge to packed conference halls. The voice can be affected by smoke, poor air quality, overuse, allergies, or infections. Ginger has long been touted as an effective home remedy for vocal issues and is widely used by many performers today. It has the ability to lower levels of prostaglandins and leukotrienes in the body that cause inflammation and subsequent pain from compressed nerves of the vocal cords. This will improve any hoarseness and return the quality of the voice to normal.

If the irritation is from a virus or bacteria, ginger is a strong remedy to rid the body of infections from these sources. It will aid the immune system in destroying the germs more quickly and allow the vocal tissues to heal. Ginger also has warming properties and can increase blood flow to the area. This improves tone and vocal flexibility. Drinking ginger tea maintains healthy tissue in the vocal cords and provides hydration to thin any phlegm that may impede performance. Before heading out for karaoke with friends, sip a ginger concoction, and the vocal cords will be in peak condition.

CHAPTER 3

FOR THE COSMETICIAN IN YOU

NUTRITION

HEALTH

COSMETICS

BEAUTIFUL SKIN

82. ACNE

Having clear skin gives us confidence to face fears, take risks, and reach for goals. Waking up on the morning of a big presentation in front of a hundred colleagues and seeing acne has erupted across the chin can really make a person feel self-conscious, anxious, or even depressed. Acne is a skin condition that results in pimples, blackheads, whiteheads, cysts, nodules, and papules. It often appears on the face, but it can also show up on the neck, chest, back, upper arms, shoulders, and buttocks. Acne is the most common skin problem in the United States. It happens when dead skin cells stick together with sebum (oil) and become trapped inside the pore. Bacteria living on the skin can sometimes get stuck in the pores with the dead skin cells. This provides a perfect breeding ground for them, and they quickly multiply. The skin becomes inflamed. If the acne goes deeper into the skin, a nodule or cyst forms. Typically, acne appears in teenagers and young adults, but it can affect anyone, even babies. Scars and dark spots on the skin can result. Mild acne can be treated with over-the-counter products that contain benzoyl peroxide or salicylic acid. It takes four to eight weeks of using the product for acne to clear. For best results, a dermatologist should treat more severe cases. Prescription-grade topical treatments, whole body treatments like antibiotics, or office procedures involving lasers, lights, or chemicals may be used.

Ginger has a number of mechanisms that help keep the skin clear, smooth, and acne-free. It lowers levels of prostaglandins and leukotrienes in the body that cause inflammation and subsequent pain from compressed nerves. This helps reduce the swelling, redness, and pain associated with large, rounded blemishes. They become less noticeable and bothersome to the individual. The antibacterial properties of ginger destroy bacteria trapped in the pores to shorten the duration of the acne and support the immune system in fighting these germs. When antibiotics are prescribed, ginger may be supplemented alongside them to provide extra bacteria-fighting power. It supports a healthy digestive system, which is especially important throughout a course of antibiotics because these destroy the good bacteria in the gut. The digestive system must be working properly to absorb all the nutrients needed for glowing skin. Ginger stimulates circulation and promotes perspiration. These actions can carry toxins away from acne sites and excrete them in sweat. Finally, ginger has potent antidepressant compounds that can help elevate mood[119] if acne is causing feelings of depression.

83. AGING

The process of getting older involves many changes in the body. Arteries stiffen, bones lose density, memory declines, skin thins, and wrinkles appear. The rate at which these processes take place varies from person to person. Genetics and illness play a role in when and how we age, but our diet and lifestyle significantly impact the process. There are many theories of aging, but the free-radical theory is growing in popularity as an explanation. It is thought that free radicals are responsible for age-related damage of cells and tissues. Free radicals are unstable molecules actively looking for an electron. They attack the nearest stable molecule and steal one of their electrons, making that molecule a free radical as well. This begins a chain reaction of creating free radicals that ultimately can destroy the cell.

The key to stopping these free radicals lies in the presence of antioxidants. Ginger contains around forty antioxidant compounds. These compounds sidle up to free radicals and give them an electron. Now they are happy and leave neighboring molecules alone. Cells and tissues continue to live, and the aging process is slowed. This happens throughout the body, from the liver to the skin. And as we've discussed, ginger stimulates circulation and promotes perspiration. These actions can carry toxins away in the blood and excrete them in sweat. Toxins are poisonous substances that promote infection and disease and accelerate aging. Removing toxins keeps tissues healthy and functioning well.

Ginger also promotes the production of collagen. Collagen gives bodies support and structure. It is a main component of skin, hair, and nails, and as collagen is lost, the signs of aging set in. Vitamin C in ginger is involved in collagen formation. Consuming ginger orally or applying it topically in creams and lotions will slow aging and give a healthier and more youthful appearance.

84. BURNS

A burn causes damage to the skin and possibly underlying tissues from sunlight, heat, chemicals, electricity, or radiation. There are three types of burns. First degree burns affect the outer layer of skin and cause minor inflammation, redness, and pain. Second degree burns damage the outer layer of skin and the layer underneath. They are characterized by blisters, redness, and pain. Third degree burns are the most serious and damage the deepest layer of skin tissue. They have a white, leathery appearance. Treatment for minor burns includes cleaning the wound, applying antibiotic cream, and taking pain medication. More severe burns should be treated by a medical professional.

Ginger can be used to replace both the antibiotic cream and the pain medication in the treatment of minor burns. This is a ready and inexpensive remedy that can be prepared at home. Ginger lowers the levels of prostaglandins and leukotrienes in the body that cause inflammation and subsequent pain. This helps reduce swelling of the burned tissue and decreases redness and pain. Ginger is also an antibacterial agent and can attack any bacteria that find their way through the damaged skin. This discourages infection and helps the immune system to heal the burn. This was demonstrated in a study of hairless rats that were pretreated with a topical application of 3 percent ginger extract for twenty-one days. Superficial abrasion wounds healed more quickly and showed increased collagen production over rats not pretreated with ginger.[120] The support structure of the burned skin is enhanced by vitamin C in ginger, which promotes collagen formation and rebuilding tissue at the site of the burn. Nutrients are delivered to the damaged tissue more quickly with the help of ginger. It increases circulation and blood flow so that the skin cells have the compounds they need to generate skin tissue.

During the healing process, scar tissue can form. Ginger applied topically to the skin directly triggers the white scar tissue cells that are unable to produce melanin to mimic their neighboring normal pigmented cells. After ginger application, the cells begin to produce melanin, and the white color of scar tissue begins to be replaced by the natural color of the skin. Ginger helps new skin tissue grow at the site of the burn, prevents infection, reduces pain and swelling, and returns white scar tissue to normal color.

85. CELLULITE

Normal fat beneath the skin can push against connective tissue and cause the skin above it to pucker. This results in a dimpled appearance of the skin that many find undesirable. It is extremely common in women and occurs most often on the hips, thighs, buttocks, and stomach. This is not just a condition for overweight people, because thin individuals can have cellulite, too. It has a strong genetic component, so if one generation had it, the next generation is likely to as well. To reduce the appearance of cellulite, stay hydrated, lose weight if needed, and exercise to tone the muscles and boost circulation to the areas.

Strong and abundant connective tissue will prevent fatty cells from bulging to the surface. Ginger helps maintain the connective tissue by stimulating circulation, which brings more nutrients to the cells to keep the tissue healthy. It also contains vitamin C, which is used in the formation and maintenance of collagen, a protein that makes connective tissue.

HOMEMADE GINGER PASTE

1 part freshly grated ginger
2 parts olive oil

1. Combine ginger and olive oil to form a paste.
2. Apply to the skin to stimulate blood flow to the area and increase nutrient availability to grow new, healthy connective tissue.
3. Make sure to rinse thoroughly afterward. Whether it's summer at the beach or sweating in the gym, ginger will have the skin looking its best.

86. CUTS AND SCRAPES

Wounding the skin is a very common occurrence and happens to everyone. Whether it's slicing the tip of the finger while dicing carrots or slipping on gravel and scraping a knee, cuts and scrapes tear the skin tissue and often cause bleeding. If the wound is deep, bleeds heavily, or has an object embedded in it, seek medical attention. If it's minor, however, it can be addressed at home. Wash your hands with soap and water. Clean the cut or scrape by pouring cool, clean water over it to remove dirt and debris. Then wash with soap and water. Once clean, an antibiotic ointment can be applied.

Here is where ginger comes in. Ginger is an antibacterial agent and can attack and kill any bacteria that find their way into an

NUTRITION

HEALTH

COSMETICS

open wound. This discourages infection and helps the immune system heal the skin. Ginger contains vitamin C, which promotes collagen formation to enhance the skin's support structure and re-build tissue at the site of injury. This was demonstrated in a study of hairless rats that were pretreated with a topical application of 3 percent ginger extract for twenty-one days. Superficial abrasion wounds healed more quickly and showed increased collagen pro-duction over rats not pretreated with ginger.[121]

Sometimes, there is pain and swelling in and around the cut. Ginger reduces these symptoms by lowering prostaglandin and leukotriene levels. The result is similar to taking ibuprofen.[122] Some cuts and scrapes heal nicely, and you may never see where they once existed. Others leave scars, forever reminding you of the inci-dent. Scars fade over time, but they never go away and are always noticeable. Ginger applied topically to the skin directly triggers white scar tissue cells to produce melanin. The white color of the scar tissue begins to be replaced by the natural color of the skin. Ginger can be applied directly to the skin (not essential ginger oil) or consumed every day in food or as a supplement to support the body during the wound healing process. (See the Homemade Ginger Paste recipe on page 96.)

87. EXFOLIATION

Exfoliating on a regular basis keeps the skin glowing and fresh and is a healthy habit to get into. The process removes dead skin cells from the outermost layer of the skin to expose the new, radiant skin underneath. This skin is smooth and soft and immediately makes a person look younger. Exfoliating is usually done by either mechanical means with a loofah, a pumice stone, a body brush, or exfoliating gloves or by chemical means at a spa or doctor's office. Most take care to exfoliate the face, but doing the entire body can make your skin feel alive and look luminous. Moreover, it allows moisturizer to penetrate deeper into the skin for better hydration.

Part of the exfoliating process is to use a facial or body scrub. There are many available in stores, but an inexpensive and very effective way to remove dead skin and start the rejuvenation process is to make a scrub at home with ginger. The ginger in the scrub will stimulate blood circulation and bring nutrients to the skin. These are necessary for the creation of healthy, new cells and to remove toxins that can make skin look sallow and old. Ginger has antibacterial properties, so any skin condition, like acne, will benefit from destruction of bacterial cells and allow the skin to heal. It's important to protect the new cells that the exfoliating process brings to the surface. Ginger does just this. It contains over forty antioxidants and can defend the skin against free radical–inflicted sun damage.

HOMEMADE GINGER EXFOLIATING SCRUB

1 tablespoon grated fresh ginger
1 tablespoon freshly squeezed lime juice
1/4 cup sea salt

1. Combine and mix all ingredients.
2. Apply to the skin and scrub gently. Rinse with warm water.

88. FRAGRANCE

Some people have an affinity for sweet smells, others like flowery scents, while still others prefer strong musky or woodsy aromas. Fortunately, there is no shortage of pleasing fragrances to suit every taste and mood. They are added to a huge array of products from cosmetics and cleaners to garbage bags and tissues. When "fragrance" or "perfume" is listed as an ingredient on a product, it more often than not is a combination of aromatic chemicals. The US Department of Health and Human Services reports that there are over five thousand different fragrance chemicals used in products. Using products with synthetic chemicals may cause dermatitis, disrupt our hormones, or even be toxic to our brains. Make sure to read the ingredients and stay away from synthetic fragrances. Finding products that use ginger essential oil for fragrance, however, will provide the benefits of a wonderfully aromatic product without the harmful side effects of synthetic fragrances. Most products using ginger for its fresh, lemon-like, and spicy notes use the essential oil from the rhizome.

Purchase ginger essential oil and combine it with other essential oils in a carrier oil to create a unique and personal perfume. Try blending ten drops of ginger essential oil with lavender and jasmine in one tablespoon of jojoba oil. Store in a dark, airtight container. This is quite concentrated, so use sparingly by dabbing a drop on the pulse points. Other combinations that work well with ginger are orange, lemon, lime, pine, nutmeg, clove, and cinnamon.

89. HYPOPIGMENTED SCARS

A thickened and permanent patch of skin that forms over a wound when the skin is injured by a cut, scrape, sore, or burn is a scar. If this skin is whiter than the normal skin tone, it is hypopigmented. These skin cells have lost the ability to produce melanin, which provides pigmentation and a darker color to the skin. Scars will fade over time, but they never go away. Some scars are small and not bothersome to the person. Others are larger or in conspicuous places like the face. These can make a person feel self-conscious or believe that it negatively impacts their physical attractiveness. There are a number of procedures available to reduce the appearance of scars. Chemical peels, dermabrasion, and laser therapy are a few. These require trips to the doctor and can be expensive. They also come with a risk of side effects, including infection, redness, pain, and bruising.

Ginger applied topically to the skin directly triggers the white scar tissue cells that are unable to produce melanin to mimic their neighboring normal pigmented cells. They begin to produce melanin, and the white scar tissue begins to be replaced by the natural color of the skin. Slice fresh ginger and rub directly over the scar so that the natural juices come out and make the scar tissue moist. The skin will absorb the juice. Do this several times a day for a period of six to twelve weeks. Improvements should begin within just a few weeks, although complete disappearance of the white scar will take longer.

90. LIP PLUMPER

Having full, pouty lips is in high fashion today. This has women (mostly) running to the doctor's office to augment their natural lip shapes. Collagen, fat injections, and implants were popular at the beginning of this trend, but hyaluronic acid is now commonly preferred. This dermal filler is injected into the lips and around the mouth to increase the volume of the lips. It is a natural substance in the body and comes with fewer side effects than the older methods. Still, though, swelling, bruising, pain at the injection site, allergies, lip irregularities, and infection can occur.

To temporarily achieve the look without the side effects or the whopping $500–$2,000 doctor's bill, try making lip plumper at home using ginger in a carrier oil with other ingredients. Fine lines will appear diminished and give a more youthful appearance. The ginger in the recipe stimulates circulation and brings more blood to the lips, opening blood vessels and creating plumper, rosier lips. The cinnamon has a similar effect on the skin and causes slight swelling and color, while the peppermint cools and soothes the skin. The coconut oil acts as a carrier for the ingredients, but it is also a wonderful moisturizer.

GINGER LIP PLUMPER

1/4 teaspoon ground ginger
1/4 teaspoon ground cinnamon
3 tablespoons melted coconut oil
2 drops essential peppermint oil

1. Mix together ginger and ground cinnamon in melted coconut oil. Add essential peppermint oil.
2. Mix thoroughly and apply to the lips for a few minutes. A slight warm, tingly sensation should be felt.
3. Rinse off. Lips will feel smoother and fuller and have a rosy appearance. Store remaining product in an airtight container in a cool, dark place.

91. REJUVENATION

Aging changes our skin. The smooth and toned texture of youth is lost, and the skin feels drier, thinner, and more fragile. Lines develop on the forehead and around the mouth, eventually forming wrinkles. A lifetime of sun exposure plays a large role in speeding up the aging of skin. The UV rays break down fibers in the skin that cause it to lose elasticity, so it stretches and sags. There are many expensive treatments like laser resurfacing and chemical peels that will remove the surface layer of skin cells to improve texture, smooth wrinkles, and reduce the look of blemishes and scars. A topical treatment with a ginger mask can have similar effects and can be done at home.

The ginger in this mask has antiaging benefits that contribute to radiant skin. It increases circulation so that more blood cells move to the surface of the skin, bringing oxygen and nutrients. These stimulate the production of new, healthy skin cells to replace the dead ones and give a fresher outward appearance. Ginger has a plumping effect on the skin, which is noticeable in older skin that has lost much of the fat deposits and has a leaner, aged look.

NUTRITION

HEALTH

COSMETICS

Wrinkles look smoother because of the plumping effect but also because ginger contains vitamin C, which promotes collagen formation that enhances support structure and firms up the skin.

Adult acne is not uncommon, and this ginger mask will help clear up acne with its antibacterial and anti-inflammatory properties, resulting in a more even and pleasing complexion. A recent study tested body cream injected with essential oils, including ginger, on twenty-nine healthy volunteers. Skin felt significantly smoother. Its use is suggested as a natural source for spa and cosmetic products to rejuvenate skin.[123]

GINGER MASK

1 part powdered ginger
1 part raw honey
1 part fresh lemon juice

1. Mix ginger, honey, and lemon juice in equal parts. Refrigerate to allow the mixture to become thicker.
2. Smooth mask over the face, taking care to avoid the eyes. Relax for twenty minutes, then rinse mask off with warm water. The skin should feel hydrated, stimulated, and smooth to the touch.

92. REMOVE SUNTAN

It used to be in vogue for people to lie outside for hours in the summer sun, even going so far as to lather the body in oil and set a timer to know when to turn over so that a consistent tan was developed. Today, however, we know more about the damaging effects of the sun's UV rays and how they contribute to skin aging and disease. Sometimes, though, sunscreen is forgotten. What can result is a partial tan on the legs, arms, and face with clear markings where the skin was covered with clothes. This is not a good look. For this reason, the person may choose to remove the suntan. In other parts of the world, tanning to darken the skin is not desirable and lighter skin is preferred. Accidental suntans are a cause of annoyance, and many seek ways to remove the tan.

In the scrub recipe below, ginger stimulates the flow of blood and nutrients to the skin to create new skin cells to replace the tanned ones that are sloughed off by the gentle abrasion of the sugar and the high citric acid content in the lemon. Vitamin E in both ginger and olive oil is used in skin regeneration and in locking in moisture to keep the skin healthy and hydrated. Ginger, olive oil, and lemon all contain antioxidants to protect the skin from the destructive rays of the sun and keep the skin cells healthy. Gently exfoliate the skin with this scrub and notice lighter, brighter, softer skin.

GINGER SUNTAN SCRUB

2 tablespoons ginger
2 tablespoons fresh lemon juice
1/2 cup olive oil
1/2 cup sugar

1. Combine ginger and lemon juice. Add olive oil and sugar. This makes a scrub to remove a suntan safely and effectively with just a few applications.

NUTRITION

HEALTH

COSMETICS

NUTRITION

HEALTH

COSMETICS

93. TONE AND MOISTURIZE

Having toned and moisturized skin gives the appearance of youth. Smooth, even texture without blemishes, dark spots, acne scars, or blotches is the hallmark of beauty, and having beautiful skin like this is something everyone desires. Living a healthy lifestyle, eating properly, and getting exercise and plenty of sleep will help achieve this. Aging, however, causes the skin to begin to sag and wrinkles to form. Skin looks dull and tired. Oftentimes, more help is needed.

Ginger stimulates collagen production to improve skin firmness and elasticity. This reduces sagging skin and the look of fine lines and wrinkles. The result is smoother, younger-looking skin. Its many antioxidants prevent free radicals from UV rays and toxins from damaging skin cells. New, healthy cells on the surface of the skin give a brighter, more radiant appearance. Any toxins present in the skin cells will be swept away more quickly by the increased blood flow through the skin tissue that ginger generates. More blood also brings more nutrients to the cells so they can regenerate and function optimally. Drinking ginger as a tea will help hydrate the skin. Also, ginger essential oil can be added to jojoba oil and applied to the face as a deep-penetrating moisturizer that doesn't clog the pores.

94. UNDEREYE PuFFINESS

As we age, the tissue around the eyes begins to lose elasticity and weaken. Fat that was once in the upper eyelid may now move to the lower eyelid. This causes a puffy appearance. The effect is compounded if fluid accumulates here, too. Over time, the skin under the eyes can look loose, saggy, dark, and swollen. This look does not bother some people, but others want to reduce this puffiness to improve their appearance. Getting enough sleep, sleeping with the head elevated, or using a cool compress under the eyes are common suggestions.

Another way to reduce puffiness is to use ginger. Ginger can be added to the diet or applied topically with cool ginger tea bags under the eyes. It increases the circulation of blood and brings nutrients to the tissues under the eyes, giving them fuel and keeping them healthy. The blood takes away toxins and other impurities that increase inflammation. Because the skin around the eyes is thinner than the rest of the body, changes in levels of inflammation are more noticeable. Ginger can decrease inflammation by lowering levels of prostaglandins and leukotrienes in the tissues, which are involved in the inflammatory response. This will shrink undereye tissue for a more natural look. To provide support to the structural integrity of the eye tissue, ginger can stimulate collagen production so that fat tissue from other areas does not fall under the eye as readily.

NUTRITION

HEALTH

COSMETICS

GORGEOUS HAIR

95. HAIR LOSS

Hair grows everywhere on the body except the palms of the hands and the soles of the feet. Countless hours and money are spent trying to get rid of hair on the body, yet every hair on the head is clung to as if it were made of gold. Healthy, shiny, lustrous hair is a sign of beauty and a point of fashion and personal expression. Hair loss is common in men, though it can happen in women and children. As excessive hair falls out and bald spots appear, a person may undergo significant anxiety and feel exposed, inadequate, or unattractive. It happens when hair follicles on the head no longer produce new hair cells. Heredity plays a large role in hair loss and affects the age it begins, the rate at which it occurs, and the pattern it takes. Medications, disease, and hormone changes may also cause excessive hair loss. To counteract hair loss, people use medications to try to stimulate growth or slow loss. Others undergo surgery and transplant tiny plugs of skin containing hairs into the scalp. These come with side effects like rapid heart rate, sexual dysfunction, pain, infection, and scarring.

Ginger is an alternative treatment that can stimulate hair growth. It increases circulation of blood to the scalp, bringing nutrients to skin cells to keep them functioning, dividing, and growing. Areas of the scalp that are patchy from hair loss can begin to grow hair once again. All this can happen without any harmful side effects.

GINGER HAIR OIL

1 part grated fresh ginger
1 part jojoba oil

1. Mix ginger and jojoba oil. Apply to the scalp and let sit for approximately 30 minutes.
2. Rinse and shampoo. Do this several times a week and begin to see results within a month.

96. CONDITION AND PROTECT

There are about 100,000 to 150,000 hairs on the human head. That is a lot of strands to take care of! Each strand of hair consists of three layers, with the outer layer, or *cuticle*, protecting the inner two layers. When the hair is healthy, the scales of the cuticle overlap tightly and protect the inner layers. When it becomes damaged, however, the scales of the cuticle loosen and separate, exposing the layers underneath. The hair looks dry and dull and may break easily. Now the inner layers can become damaged from exposure to the UV rays of the sun, heat, pollution, chlorine, or any of the array of chemicals found in hair products and treatments.

To add and lock in moisture, essential ginger oil mixed with jojoba oil can be applied directly to the hair. Ginger provides zinc and iron, both needed to create healthy hair structure. The mois-ture-rich oil of ginger combined with the jojoba oil can deeply penetrate the hair shaft to provide hydration at its core and a pro-tective barrier on the outer cuticle to lock moisture in.

97. DANDRUFF

Dandruff is a chronic condition marked by the flaking of skin cells on the scalp. They are visible as white, oily-looking flakes of skin on the hair and shoulders. It is not a dangerous condition, but it can be embarrassing for some people. Dandruff is usually worse in the fall and winter when the scalp is subjected to the drier, cooler, outdoor air and heated indoor air, which depletes moisture in the skin. It can be caused by not shampooing enough so that dead skin cells mix with oils. This causes a buildup and subsequent shedding of these cells as dandruff.

Yeast on the scalp can irritate some people and cause an over-production of skin cells, which flake off as dandruff. Dry skin can cause smaller, drier flakes to appear. One of the most common causes of dandruff is seborrheic dermatitis. This is a condition in which oily skin is covered in flaky white or yellow scales. Mild cas-es are easy to treat with daily cleansing to reduce oil and skin cell buildup. Others cases are more difficult and may need medicated shampoos. Some shampoos contain antifungal and antibacterial agents to kill the microbes. Others work by slowing the death rate of skin cells to reduce buildup and flaking.

Ginger has compounds that destroy yeast and fungal cells. The amount of itching and dandruff produced will be greatly reduced or even entirely stopped. Its anti-inflammatory compounds can reduce irritation of the scalp that cause red and tender skin, other symptoms associated with these infections.

If dry skin is the culprit, ginger can help here, too. It increases blood circulation to the scalp, nourishing and moisturizing the cells and taking away toxins. Ginger encourages a healthy rate of cell turnover so that dead skin cells are shed at a normal rate.

Ayurvedic medicine has long used ginger to treat dandruff. If the source of dandruff is yeast or the fungus causing seborrheic dermatitis, use the following recipe for relief.

GINGER DANDRUFF TREATMENT

3 drops ginger essential oil
2 tablespoons sesame seed oil

1. Mix ginger essential oil and sesame seed oil. Massage into the scalp for 10 minutes.
2. After using the ginger oil treatment, rinse the scalp and gently shampoo. Repeat this process at least three times a week to maintain results.

98. SPLIT ENDS

The outer layer of the hair shaft is called the *cuticle*. It is very strong and made up of overlapping layers of protein called *keratin*. It protects the inner layers and is what gives hair its flexibility and volume. The cuticle can become damaged from chemicals,

NUTRITION

UV rays, chlorine, heat, or physical stress such as frequent, vigorous brushing or use of hair extensions. When the cuticle becomes damaged, it can no longer hold the hair shaft together and splits. Split ends give the appearance of a dry, brittle, frizzy, or untamed mane.

An herbal solution made with freshly chopped ginger and avocado oil can be applied to the ends of hair to prevent split ends. This infusion adds moisture to the hair from the combination of both oils and creates a protective barrier to lock in hydration.

GINGER HAIR MASK

2 inches fresh ginger
1/4 cup avocado oil

1. Chop ginger and place in a double boiler. Add avocado oil.
2. Heat over medium-low heat for 20 minutes, encouraging the oils from the ginger to seep into the avocado oil. Avocado oil is very heat stable, and this method will not change any of the properties of the oil.
3. Cool the mixture to room temperature and apply directly onto the ends of the hair. Leave on for 15 minutes and then rinse off. This tonic provides smooth, hydrated hair with the added benefit of amazing shine.

HEALTH

COSMETICS

STUNNING NAILS

99. NAIL FUNGUS

Fungal infections are extremely common and can infect any part of the body. When fungus targets the fingernails or toenails, white or yellow spots may begin to appear. These spots then merge to form patches and spread out. The nails become thicker, brittle, or discolored, and the edges start to crumble. The symptoms occur slowly and may eventually result in the nail detaching from the skin and falling off.

Fungal infections can actually be a sign of candida overgrowth in the body. *Candida albicans* is a very common fungus in humans and can grow out of control in people with weakened or compromised immune systems. The good bacteria in the gut cannot compete with candida, and a systemic invasion may begin, which can show up as a fungal infection of the nails. Over-the-counter treatments are available, but they are not always effective and the chance of reoccurrence is high. Prescribed oral antifungal drugs can be used that allow new growth of the nail to be fungus-free. This is a slow process and may cause a variety of side effects from a skin rash to liver disease. Medicated polishes and creams are used, but these can take a year to get rid of the fungus. The nail can also be surgically removed, but it grows back slowly.

Ginger is a known antifungal agent and can be used topically or orally in the treatment of fungal infections. Laboratory studies on the effects of ginger extracts on *Candida albicans* show that it significantly reduces[124] or eliminates the fungus and lowers the amount of endotoxins the fungus produces.[125] Ginger's effectiveness is twofold; it can be used directly on the nail to eliminate the fungus, and it can be used within the body to help elevate the good bacteria in the gut and keep candida from overgrowing and causing infection. The nail fungus will be gone, and reoccurrence is unlikely. Add ginger to your diet and apply fresh ginger paste to the affected nail. Regular use will clear the infection.

100. STRENGTHEN NAILS

Nails are made of dead skin cells and are similar to hair in that they are mostly made up of the protein keratin. Having strong, shiny nails is a sign of health and vitality. Artificial nails and nail polish can hide natural nails, which can look and feel dull and brittle when unadorned. They can have spots, striations, bow lines, grooves, or streaks or be pale, yellow, or red rather than the normal pinkish hue. Weak nails can be an indicator of a person's overall health, and many of the problems stem from poor function of the digestive tract.

Ginger supports the digestive system to ensure adequate nutrients are absorbed from food and toxins are eliminated. Seventy percent of the immune system is in the gut. A healthy gut equates to a healthy immune system, and healthy bodies grow beautiful nails. Nutrition is highly important for the development of strong nails, and ginger can provide many of the essential nutrients required. If the nails have ridges, more magnesium is needed. If there are white spots, eat more zinc. Brittle nails require more calcium, and spoon-shaped nails can be improved with iron. Consuming ginger in the diet will also increase the supply of antioxidants ready to protect the body from oxidative stress, which is felt in every cell of the body, including new nail cells. Preventative care now will ensure your nails will grow beautifully and be less prone to problems.

101. YELLOW STAINS

Yellow nails can result from different infections and conditions, but the most common cause is fungal infection. Some bacterial infections can turn nails yellow, as can smoking, excessive use of nail color, allergies, or disease such as yellow nail syndrome. Changes in grooming and lifestyle habits (looking at you, cigarettes) can allow new nails to grow without discoloration. Unknown causes should be explored medically.

While these suggestions will help prevent yellow nails in the future, treating yellow nails now can be done with ginger. If the cause is fungal, ginger can remove the yellow stain. There are antifungal compounds in ginger that will eliminate the fungus.[126] It can be used directly on the nail as a paste, and it can be ingested for use within the body. Regular use will clear the infection. It helps elevate the good bacteria in the gut, which prevents fungal overgrowth. The nail fungus will be gone, and a reoccurrence is unlikely because the source of infection is eliminated. The immune system will function better to prevent future fungal overgrowth. Bacterial

NUTRITION

HEALTH

COSMETICS

sources of yellow nails can be treated in the same way through ginger's antibacterial compounds. If the source of yellowing is due to physical stress, such as too-frequent nail coloring or smoking, then soaking the nails in ginger ale for ten minutes a day for a week will bleach the nails, making them bright and clean looking.

NOTES

1. Zick, S. M., Z. Djuric, and M. T. Ruffin, et al., eds. 2008. "Pharmacokinetics of [6]-gingerol, [8]-gingerol, [10]-gingerol, and [6]-shogaol and conjugate metabolites in healthy human subjects." *Cancer Epidemiology, Biomarkers, & Prevention* 17 (8): 1930–6.
2. Dioscorides, Pedanius. *De Materia Medica*. Johannesburg, South Africa: Ibidis Press, 2000.
3. Kawamoto, Y., Y. Ueno, E. Nakahashi, M. Obayashi, K. Sugihara, S. Qiao, M. Iida, M. Y. Kumasaka, I. Yajima, Y. Goto, N. Ohgami, M. Kato, and K. Takeda. 2016. "Prevention of allergic rhinitis by ginger and the molecular basis of immunosuppression by 6-gingerol through T cell inactivation." *Journal of Nutritional Biochemistry* 27 (January): 112–22.
4. Moon, M., H. G. Kim, J. G. Choi, H. Oh, P. K. Lee, S. K. Ha, S. Y. Kim, Y. Park, Y. Huh, and M. S. Oh. 2014. "6-Shogaol, an active constituent of ginger, attenuates neuroinflammation and cognitive deficits in animal models of dementia." *Biochemical and Biophysical Research Communities* 449 (1): 8–13.
5. Ghayur, M. N., A. H. Gilani, and L. J. Janssen. 2008. "Ginger attenuates acetylcholine-induced contraction and Ca2+ signalling in murine airway smooth muscle cells." *Canadian Journal of Physiology and Pharmacology* 86 (5): 264–71.
6. Townsend, Elizabeth A., Matthew E. Siviski, Yi Zhang, Carrie Xu, Bhupinder Hoonjan, and Charles W. Emala. 2013. "Effects of ginger and its constituents on airway smooth muscle relaxation and calcium regulation." *American Journal of Respiratory Cell and Molecular Biology* 48 (2): 157–63.
7. Alizadeh-Navaei, R., F. Roozbeh, M. Saravi, M. Pouramir, F. Jalali, and A. A. Moghadamnia. 2008. "Investigation of the effect of ginger on the lipid levels: a double blind controlled clinical trial." *Saudi Medical Journal* 29 (9): 1280–4.
8. Liu, Rongxia, Elke H. Heiss, Nadine Sider, Andreas Schinkovitz, Barbara Gröblacher, Dean Guo, Franz Bucar, Rudolf Bauer, Verena M. Dirsch, and Atanas G. Atanasov. 2015. "Identification and characterization of [6]-shogaol from ginger as inhibitor of vascular smooth muscle cell proliferation." *Molecular Nutrition & Food Research* 59 (5): 843–52.
9. Koo, K. L, A. J. Ammit, V. H. Tran, C. C. Duke, and B. D. Roufogalis. 2001. "Gingerols and related analogues inhibit arachidonic acid-induced human

platelet serotonin release and aggregation." *Thrombosis Research* 103 (5): 387–97.

10. Nurtjahja-Tjendraputra, E., A. J. Ammit, B. D. Roufogalis, V. H. Tran, and C. C. Duke. 2003. "Effective anti-platelet and COX-1 enzyme inhibitors from pungent constituents of ginger." *Thrombosis Research* 111 (4–5): 259–65.

11. Young, H. Y., J. C. Liao, Y. S. Chang, Y. L. Luo, M. C. Lu, and W. H. Peng. 2006. "Synergistic effect of ginger and nifedipine on human platelet aggregation: a study in hypertensive patients and normal volunteers." *American Journal of Chinese Medicine* 34 (4): 545–51.

12. Elkady, A. I., O. A. Abuzinadah, N. A Baeshen, and T. R. Rahmy. 2012. "Differential control of growth, apoptotic activity, and gene expression in human breast cancer cells by extracts derived from medicinal herbs Zingiber officinale." *Journal of Biomedicine and Biotechnology* 2012: 614356.

13. Ghayur, "Ginger attenuates acetylcholine-induced contraction and Ca2+ signalling in murine airway smooth muscle cells."

14. Townsend, "Effects of ginger and its constituents on airway smooth muscle relaxation and calcium regulation."

15. Azvolinsky, Anna. "Ginger Root Extract's Potential in Colorectal Cancer Prevention." CancerNetwork.com, October 25, 2011. http://www.cancernetwork.com/colorectal-cancer/ginger-root-extract's-potential-colorectal-cancer-prevention.

16. Manju, V., and N. Nalini. 2005. "Chemopreventive efficacy of ginger, a naturally occurring anticarcinogen during the initiation, post-initiation stages of 1, 2 dimethylhydrazine-induced colon cancer." *Clinica Chimica Acta* 358 (1–2): 60–7.

17. Pan, M. H., M. C. Hsieh, J. M. Kuo, C. S. Lai, H. Wu, S. Sang, and C. T. Ho. 2008. "[6]-shogaol induces apoptosis in human colorectal carcinoma cells via ROS production, caspase activation, and GADD 153 expression." *Molecular Nutrition & Food Research* 52 (5): 527–37.

18. Brown, A. C., C. Shah, J. Liu, J. T. Pham, J. G. Zhang, and M. R. Jadus. 2009. "Ginger's (Zingiber officinale Roscoe) inhibition of rat colonic adenocarcinoma cells proliferation and angiogenesis in vitro." *Phytotherapy Research* 23 (5): 640–5.

19. Mozaffari-Khosravi, H., B. Talaei, B. A. Jalali, A. Najarzadeh, and M. R. Mozayan. 2014. "The effect of ginger powder supplementation on insulin resistance and glycemic indices in patients with type 2 diabetes: a randomized, double-blind, placebo-controlled trial." *Complementary Therapies in Medicine* 22 (1): 9–16.

20. Kadnur, S. V., and R. K. Goyal. 2005. "Beneficial effects of Zingiber officinale Roscoe on fructose induced hyperlipidemia and hyperinsulinemia in rats."

Indian Journal of Experimental Biology 43 (12): 1161–4.

21. Islam, M. S., and H. Choi. 2008. "Comparative effects of dietary ginger (Zingiber officinale) and garlic (Allium sativum) investigated in a type 2 diabetes model of rats." *Journal of Medicinal Food* 11 (1): 152–9.

22. Ishiguro, K., T. Ando, O. Maeda, N. Ohmiya, Y. Niwa, K. Kadomatsu, and H. Goto. 2007. "Ginger ingredients reduce viability of gastric cancer cells via distinct mechanisms." *Biochemical and Biophysical Research Communities* 362 (1): 218–23.

23. Alizadeh-Navaei, R., "Investigation of the effect of ginger on the lipid levels."

24. Wang, C. C., L. G. Chen, L. T. Lee, and L. L. Yang. 2007. "Effects of [6]-gingerol, an antioxidant from ginger, on inducing apoptosis in human leukemic HL-60 cells." *In Vivo* 17 (6): 641–5.

25. Liu, Qun, Yong-Bo Peng, Ping Zhou, Lian-Wen Qi, Mu Zhang, Ning Gao, E-Hu Liu, and Ping Li. 2013. "6-Shogaol induces apoptosis in human leukemia cells through a process involving caspase-mediated cleavage of eIF2α." *Molecular Cancer* 12: 135.

26. Chen C. Y., T. Z. Liu, Y. W. Liu, et al., eds. 2007. "[6]-shogaol (alkanone from ginger) induces apoptotic cell death of human hepatoma p53 mutant Mahlavusubline via an oxidative stress-mediated caspase-dependent mechanism." *Journal of Agricultural and Food Chemistry* 55 (3): 948–54.

27. Atta, A. H., T. A. Elkoly, S. M. Mouneir, G. Kamel, N. A. Alwabel, and S. Zaher. 2010. "Hepatoprotective Effect of Methanol Extracts of Zingiber officinale and Cichorium intybus." *Indian Journal of Pharmaceutical Science* 72 (5): 564–70.

28. Sahebkar, Amirhossein. 2011. "Potential efficacy of ginger as a natural supplement for nonalcoholic fatty liver disease." *World Journal of Gastroenterology* 17 (2): 271–2.

29. Mallikarjuna, K., P. Sahitya Chetan, K. Sathyavelu Reddy, and W. Rajendra. 2008. "Ethanol toxicity: Rehabilitation of hepatic antioxidant defense system with dietary ginger." *Fitoterapia* 79 (3): 174–8.

30. Wigler, I., I. Grotto, D. Caspi, and M. Yaron. 2003. "The effects of Zintona EC (a ginger extract) on symptomatic gonarthritis." *Osteoarthritis Cartilage* 11: 783–9.

31. Altman, R. D., and K. C. Marcussen. 2001. "Effects of ginger extract on knee pain in patients with osteoarthritis." *Arthritis & Rheumatology* 44: 2531–8.

32. Haghighi, M., A. Khalva, T. Toliat, and S. Jallaei. 2005. "Comparing the effects of ginger (Zingiber officinale) extract and ibuprofen on patients with osteoarthritis." *Archives of Iranian Medicine* 8: 267–71.

33. Sung, B., A. Murakami, B. O. Oyajobi, and B. B. Aggarwal. 2009. "Zerumbone abolishes RANKL-induced NF-kappaB activation, inhibits

osteoclastogenesis, and suppresses human breast cancer-induced bone loss in athymic nude mice." *Cancer Research* 69 (4): 1477–84.

34. Rhode, J., S. Fogoros, S. Zick, H. Wahl, K. A. Griffith, J. Huang, and J. R. Liu. 2007. "Ginger inhibits cell growth and modulates angiogenic factors in ovarian cancer cells." *BMC Complementary and Alternative Medicine* 7: 44.

35. Park, Y. J., J. Wen, S. Bang, S. W. Park, and S. Y. Song. 2006. "[6]-gingerol induces cell cycle arrest and cell death of mutant p53-expressing pancreatic cancer cells." *Yonsei Medical Journal* 47 (5): 688–97.

36. Zhang, S., Q. Liu, Y. Liu, H. Qiao, and Y. Liu. 2012. "Zerumbone, a Southeast Asian Ginger Sesquiterpene, Induced Apoptosis of Pancreatic Carcinoma Cells through p53 Signaling Pathway." *Evidence-Based Complementary and Alternative Medicine* 2012: 936030.

37. Kabuto, H., M. Nishizawa, M. Tada, C. Higashio, T. Shishibori, and M. Kohno. 2005. "Zingerone [4-(4-hydroxy-3-methoxyphenyl)-2-butanone] prevents 6-hydroxydopamine-induced dopamine depression in mouse striatum and increases superoxide scavenging activity in serum." *Neurochemical Research* 30 (3): 325–32.

38. Karna, P., S. Chagani, S. R. Gundala, P. C. Rida, G. Asif, V. Sharma, M. V. Gupta, and R. Aneja. 2012. "Benefits of whole ginger extract in prostate cancer." *British Journal of Nutrition* 107 (4): 473–84.

39. Kurapati, Kesava Rao V., Thangavel Samikkannu, Dakshayani B. Kadiyala, Saiyed M. Zainulabedin, Nimisha Gandhi, Sadhana S. Sathaye, Manohar A. Indap, Nawal Boukli, Jose W. Rodriguez, and Madhavan P. N. Nair. 2012. "Combinatorial cytotoxic effects of Curcuma longa and Zingiber officinale on the PC-3M prostate cancer cell line." *Journal of Basic Clinical Physiology and Pharmacology* 23 (4): 139–146.

40. Uz, E., O. F. Karatas, E. Mete, R. Bayrak, O. Bayrak, A. F. Atmaca, O. Atis, M. E. Yildirim, and A. Akcay. 2009. "The effect of dietary ginger (Zingiber officinals Rosc) on renal ischemia/reperfusion injury in rat kidneys." *Renal Failure* 31 (4): 25–160.

41. M. F. Mahmoud, A. A. Diaai, and F. Ahmed. 2012. "Evaluation of the efficacy of ginger, Arabic gum, and Boswellia in acute and chronic renal failure." *Renal Failure* 34 (1): 73–82.

42. Srivastava, K. C., and T. Mustafa. 1992. "Ginger (Zingiber officinale) in rheumatism and musculoskeletal disorders." *Medical Hypotheses* 39 (4): 342–8.

43. Tripathi, S., K. G. Maier, D. Bruch, and D. S. Kittur. 2007. "Effect of [6]-gingerol on pro-inflammatory cytokine production and costimulatory molecule expression in murine peritoneal macrophages." *Journal of Surgical Research* 138 (2): 209–13.

44. Nigam, N., K. Bhui, S. Prasad, J. George, and Y. Shukla. 2009. "[6]-gingerol induces reactive oxygen species regulated mitochondrial cell death pathway in humanepidermoid carcinoma A431 cells." *Chemico-Biological Interactions* 181: 77–84.

45. Chung, W. Y., Y. J. Jung, Y. J. Surh, S. S. Lee, and K. K. Park. 2001. "Antioxidative and antitumor promoting effects of [6]-paradol and its homologs." *Mutation Research* 496 (1–2): 199–206.

46. El-Abhar, H. S., L. N. Hammad, and H. S. Gawad. 2008. "Modulating effect of ginger extract on rats with ulcerative colitis." *Journal of Ethnopharmacology* 118 (3): 367–72.

47. Uz Zaman, Sameer, Mrutyunjay M. Mirje, and S. Ramabhimaiah. 2014. "Evaluation of the anti-ulcerogenic effect of Zingiber officinale (Ginger) root in rats." *International Journal of Current Microbiology and Applied Sciences* 3 (1): 347–54.

48. Nanjundaiah, Siddaraju M., Harish Nayaka Mysore Annaiah, and Shylaja M. Dharmesh. 2011. "Gastroprotective Effect of Ginger Rhizome (Zingiber officinale) Extract: Role of Gallic Acid and Cinnamic Acid in H+, K+-ATPase/H. pylori Inhibition and Anti-Oxidative Mechanism." *Evidence-Based Complementary and Alternative Medicine* 2011 (2): 249487.

49. Bera, K., G. Nosalova, V. Sivova, and B. Ray. 2016. "Structural Elements and Cough Suppressing Activity of Polysaccharides from Zingiber officinale Rhizome." *Phytotherapy Research* 30 (1): 105–11.

50. Wu, K. L., C. K. Rayner, S. K. Chuah, et al., eds. 2008. "Effects of ginger on gastric emptying and motility in healthy humans." *European Journal of Gastroenterology and Hepatology* 20 (5): 436–40.

51. Yamahara, J., Q. R. Huang, Y. H. Li, L. Xu, and H. Fujimura. 1990. "Gastrointestinal motility enhancing effect of ginger and its active constituents." *Chemical and Pharmaceutical Bulletin* 38 (2): 430–1.

52. Gupta, Y. K., and M. Sharma. 2001. "Reversal of pyrogallol-induced delay in gastric emptying in rats by ginger (Zingiber officinale)." *Methods and Findings in Experimental and Clinical Pharmacology* 23 (9): 501–3.

53. Bera, "Structural Elements and Cough Suppressing Activity of Polysaccharides from Zingiber officinale Rhizome."

54. Deng, X. Y., J. S. Xue, H. Y. Li, Z. Q. Ma, Q. Fu, R. Qu, and S. P. Ma. 2015. "Geraniol produces antidepressant-like effects in a chronic unpredictable mild stress mice model." *Physiology & Behavior* 152 (Pt A): 264–71.

55. Martinez, D. M., A. Barcellos, A. M. Casaril, L. Savegnago, and E. J. Lernardão. 2014. "Antidepressant-like activity of dehydrozingerone: involvement of the serotonergic and noradrenergic systems." *Pharmacology Biochemistry and Behavior* 127: 111–17.

56. Wang, X., W. Jia, A. Zhao, and X. Wang. 2006. "Anti-influenza agents from plants and traditional Chinese medicine." *Phytotherapy Research* 20 (5): 335–41.

57. Dyab, A. K., D. A. Yones, Z. Z. Ibraheim, and T. M. Hassan. 2016. "Anti-giardial therapeutic potential of dichloromethane extracts of Zingiber officinale and Curcuma longa in vitro and in vivo." *Parasitology Research* 115 (7): 2637–45.

58. Suekawa, M., A. Ishige, K. Yuasa, K. Sudo, M. Aburada, and E. Hosoya. 1984. "Pharmacological studies on ginger. I. Pharmacological actions of pungent constituents, (6)-gingerol and (6)-shogaol." *Journal of Pharmacobiodynamics* 7 (11): 836–48.

59. Wu, "Effects of ginger on gastric emptying and motility in healthy humans."

60. Mahyari, S., B. Mahyari, S. A. Emami, B. Malaekeh-Nikouei, S. P. Jahanbakhsh, A. Sahebkar, and A. H. Mohammadpour. 2016. "Evaluation of the efficacy of a polyherbal mouthwash containing Zingiber officinale, Rosmarinus officinalis and Calendula officinalis extracts in patients with gingivitis: A randomized double-blind placebo-controlled trial." *Complementary Therapies in Clinical Practice* 22: 93–8.

61. Maghbooli, M., F. Golipour, A. Moghimi Esfandabadi, and M. Yousefi. 2014. "Comparison between the efficacy of ginger and sumatriptan in the ablative treatment of the common migraine." *Phytotherapy Research* 28 (3): 412–5.

62. Cady, R. K., J. Goldstein, R. Nett, R. Mitchell, M. E. Beach, and R. Browning. 2011. "A double-blind placebo-controlled pilot study of sublingual feverfew and ginger (LipiGesic™ M) in the treatment of migraine." *Headache* 51 (7): 1078–86.

63. Siddaraju, M. N., and S. M. Dharmesh. 2007. "Inhibition of gastric H+, K+-ATPase and Helicobacter pylori growth by phenolic antioxidants of Zingiber officinale." *Molecular Nutrition & Food Research* 51 (3): 324–32.

64. Drozdov, V. N., V. A. Kim, E. V. Tkachenko, and G. G. Varvanina. 2012. "Influence of a specific ginger combination on gastropathy conditions in patients with osteoarthritis of the knee or hip." *Journal of Alternative and Complementary Medicine* 18 (6): 583–8.

65. Yamahara, J., M. Mochizuki, H. Q. Rong, H. Matsuda, and H. Fujimura. 1988. "The anti-ulcer effect in rats of ginger constituents." *Journal of Ethnopharmacology* 23 (2–3): 299–304.

66. Ghayur, M. N., and A. H. Gilani. 2005. "Pharmacological basis for the medicinal use of ginger in gastrointestinal disorders." *Digestive Diseases and Sciences* 50 (10): 1889–97.

67. Yamahara, "Gastrointestinal motility enhancing effect of ginger and its active constituents."

68. Gupta, "Reversal of pyrogallol-induced delay in gastric emptying in rats by ginger (Zingiber officinale)."

69. Hu, M. L., C. K. Rayner, K. L. Wu, S. K. Chuah, W. C. Tai, Y. P. Chou, Y. C. Chiu, K. W. Chiu, and T. H. Hu. 2011. "Effect of ginger on gastric motility and symptoms of functional dyspepsia." *World Journal of Gastroenterology* 17 (1): 105–10.

70. Sahib, A. S. 2013. "Treatment of irritable bowel syndrome using a selected herbal combination of Iraqi folk medicines." *Journal of Ethnopharmacology* 148 (3): 1008–12.

71. Ghayur, "Ginger attenuates acetylcholine-induced contraction and Ca2+ signalling in murine airway smooth muscle cells."

72. Wu, "Effects of ginger on gastric emptying and motility in healthy humans."

73. Gupta, "Reversal of pyrogallol-induced delay in gastric emptying in rats by ginger."

74. Lamxay, Vichith, Hugo J. de Boer, and Lars Björk. 2011. "Traditions and plant use during pregnancy, childbirth and postpartum recovery by the Kry ethnic group in Lao PDR." *Journal of Ethnobiology and Ethnomedicine* 7: 14.

75. Ghayur, "Ginger attenuates acetylcholine-induced contraction and Ca2+ signalling in murine airway smooth muscle cells."

76. Ozgoli, G., M. Goli, and F. Moattar. 2009. "Comparison of effects of ginger, mefenamic acid, and ibuprofen on pain in women with primary dysmenorrhea." *Journal of Alternative and Complementary Medicine* 15: 129–32.

77. Rahnama, Parvin, Ali Montazeri, Hassan Fallah Huseini, Saeed Kianbakht, and Mohsen Naseri. 2012. "Effect of Zingiber officinale R. rhizomes (ginger) on pain relief in primary dysmenorrhea: a placebo randomized trial." *BMC Complementary and Alternative Medicine* 12: 92.

78. Willetts, K. E., A. Ekangaki, and J. A. Eden. 2003. "Effect of a ginger extract on pregnancy-induced nausea: a randomised controlled trial." *Australia and New Zealand Journal of Obstetrics and Gynaecology* 43 (2): 139–44.

79. Vutyavanich, T., T. Kraisarin, and R. Ruangsri. 2001. "Ginger for nausea and vomiting in pregnancy: randomized, double-masked, placebo-controlled trial." *Obstetrics and Gynecology* 97 (4): 577–82.

80. Pongrojpaw, D., C. Somprasit, and A. Chanthasenanont. 2007. "A randomized comparison of ginger and dimenhydrate in the treatment of nausea and vomiting in pregnancy." *Journal of the Medical Association of Thailand* 90 (9): 1703–9.

81. Mowrey, D. B., and D. E. Clayson. 1982. "Motion sickness, ginger, and psychophysics." *Lancet* 1 (8273): 655–7.

82. Grontved, A., T. Brask, J. Kambskard, and E. Hentzer. 1988. "Ginger root against seasickness: a controlled trial on the open sea." *Acta Oto-Laryngolica* 105 (1–2): 45–9.

83. Lien, H. C., W. M. Sun, Y. H. Chen, H. Kim, W. Hasler, and C. Owyang. 2003. "Effects of ginger on motion sickness and gastric slow-wave

dysrhythmias induced by circular vection." *American Journal of Physiolology: Gastrointestinal and Liver Physiology* 284 (3): G481–9.

84. Black, C. D., M. P. Herring, D. J. Hurley, and P. J. O'Connor. 2010. "Ginger (Zingiber officinale) reduces muscle pain caused by eccentric exercise." *Journal of Pain* 11 (9): 894–903.

85. Ryan, J. L., C. E. Heckler, J. A. Roscoe, S. R. Dakhil, J. Kirshner, P. J. Flynn, J. T. Hickok, and G. R. Morrow. 2012. "Ginger (Zingiber officinale) reduces acute chemotherapy-induced nausea: a URCC CCOP study of 576 patients." *Supportive Care in Cancer* 20 (7): 1479–89.

86. Pillai, A. K., K. K. Sharma, Y. K. Gupta, and S. Bakhshi. 2011. "Antiemetic effect of ginger powder versus placebo as an add-on therapy in children and young adults receiving high emetogenic chemotherapy." *Pediatric Blood & Cancer* 56 (2): 234–8.

87. Dabaghzadeh, F., H. Khalili, S. Dashti-Khavidaki, L. Abbasian, and A. Moeinifard. 2014. "Ginger for prevention of antiretroviral-induced nausea and vomiting: a randomized clinical trial." *Expert Opinion on Drug Safety* 13 (7): 859–66.

88. Pongrojpaw, D., and C. Chiamchanya. 2003. "The efficacy of ginger in prevention of post-operative nausea and vomiting after outpatient gynecological laparoscopy." *Journal of the Medical Association of Thailand* 86 (3): 244–50.

89. Nanthakomon, T., and D. Pongrojpaw. 2006. "The efficacy of ginger in prevention of postoperative nausea and vomiting after major gynecologic surgery." *Journal of the Medical Association of Thailand* 89 (Suppl. 4): S130–6.

90. Chaiyakunapruk, N., N. Kitikannakorn, S. Nathisuwan, K. Leeprakobboon, and C. Leelasettagool. 2006. "The efficacy of ginger for the prevention of postoperative nausea and vomiting: a meta-analysis." *American Journal of Obstetrics & Gynecology* 194 (1): 95–9.

91. Geiger, J. 2005. "The essential oil of ginger, *Zingiber officinale*, and anaesthesia." *International Journal of Aromatherapy* 15 (1): 7–14.

92. Jagetia, G. C., M. S. Baliga, P. Venkatesh, and J. N. Ulloor. 2003. "Influence of ginger rhizome (Zingiber officinale Rosc) on survival, glutathione and lipid peroxidation in mice after whole-body exposure to gamma radiation." *Radiation Research* 160 (5): 584–92.

93. Kim, J. K., Y. Kim, K. M. Na, Y. J. Surh, and T. Y. Kim. 2007. "[6]-gingerol prevents UVB-induced ROS production and COX-2 expression in vitro and in vivo." *Free Radical Research* 41 (5): 603–14.

94. Hursel, R., and M. S. Westerterp-Plantenga. 2010. "Thermogenic ingredients and body weight regulation. *International Journal of Obesity* 34 (4): 659–69.

95. Mansour, Muhammad S., Yu-Ming Ni, Amy L. Roberts, Michael Kelleman, Arindam Roychoudhury, and Marie-Pierre St-Onge. 2012. "Ginger

consumption enhances the thermic effect of food and promotes feelings of satiety without affecting metabolic and hormonal parameters in overweight men: a pilot study." *Metabolism* 61 (10): 1347–52.

96. Eldershaw, T. P., E. Q. Colquhoun, K. A. Dora, Z. C. Peng, and M. G. Clark. 1992. "Pungent principles of ginger (Zingiber officinale) are thermogenic in the perfused rat hind limb." *International Journal of Obesity and Related Metabolic Disorders* 16 (10): 755–63.

97. Bera, "Structural Elements and Cough Suppressing Activity of Polysaccharides from Zingiber officinale Rhizome."

98. Lamxay, "Traditions and plant use during pregnancy, childbirth and postpartum recovery by the Kry ethnic group in Lao PDR."

99. Ozgoli, "Comparison of effects of ginger, mefenamic acid, and ibuprofen on pain in women with primary dysmenorrhea."

100. Ibid.

101. Maghbooli, "Comparison between the efficacy of ginger and sumatriptan in the ablative treatment of the common migraine."

102. Cady, "A double-blind placebo-controlled pilot study of sublingual feverfew and ginger (LipiGesic™ M) in the treatment of migraine."

103. Hursel, "Thermogenic ingredients and body weight regulation."

104. Mansour, "Ginger consumption enhances the thermic effect of food and promotes feelings of satiety without affecting metabolic and hormonal parameters in overweight men."

105. Iwasaki, Y., A. Morita, T. Iwasawa, K. Kobata, Y. Sekiwa, Y. Morimitsu, K. Kubota, and T. Watanabe. 2006. "A nonpungent component of steamed ginger-[10]-shogaol-increases adrenaline secretion via the activation of TRPV1." *Nutritional Neuroscience* 9 (3–4): 169–78.

106. Grady, Cheryl L., Mellanie V. Springer, Donaya Hongwanishkul, Anthony R. McIntosh, and Gordon Winocur. 2006. "Age-Related Changes in Brain Activity across the Adult Lifespan." *Journal of Cognitive Neuroscience* 18 (2): 227–41.

107. Saenghong, N., J. Wattanathorn, S. Muchimapura, T. Tongun, N. Piyavhatkul, C. Banchonglikitkul, and T. Kajsongkram. 2012. "Zingiber Officinale Improves Cognitive Function of the Middle-Aged Healthy Women." *Evidence-Based Complementary and Alternative Medicine* 2012: 383062.

108. Iwasaki, "A nonpungent component of steamed ginger-[10]-shogaol-increases adrenaline secretion via the activation of TRPV1."

109. Hursel, "Thermogenic ingredients and body weight regulation."

110. Mansour, "Ginger consumption enhances the thermic effect of food and promotes feelings of satiety without affecting metabolic and hormonal parameters in overweight men."

111. Deng, "Geraniol produces antidepressant-like effects in a chronic unpredictable mild stress mice model."

112. Martinez, "Antidepressant-like activity of dehydrozingerone."

113. Wu, "Effects of ginger on gastric emptying and motility in healthy humans."

114. Yamahara, "Gastrointestinal motility enhancing effect of ginger and its active constituents."

115. Gupta, "Reversal of pyrogallol-induced delay in gastric emptying in rats by ginger (Zingiber officinale)."

116. Black, "Ginger (Zingiber officinale) reduces muscle pain caused by eccentric exercise."

117. Atashaka, Sirvan, Maghsoud Peerib, Mohammad Ali Azarbayjanib, and Stephen R. Stannard. 2014. "Effects of ginger (*Zingiber officinale Roscoe*) supplementation and resistance training on some blood oxidative stress markers in obese men." *Journal of Exercise Science & Fitness* 12 (1): 26–30.

118. Eldershaw, "Pungent principles of ginger (Zingiber officinale) are thermogenic in the perfused rat hind limb."

119. Martinez, "Antidepressant-like activity of dehydrozingerone."

120. Bhagavathula, Narasimharao, Roscoe L. Warner, Marissa DaSilva, Shannon D. McClintock, Adam Barron, Muhammad N. Aslam, Kent J. Johnson, and James Varani. 2009. "A combination of curcumin and ginger extract improves abrasion wound healing in corticosteroid-damaged hairless rat skin." *Wound Repair and Regeneration* 17 (3): 360.

121. Ibid.

122. Haghighi, "Comparing the effects of ginger (Zingiber officinale) extract and ibuprofen on patients with osteoarthritis."

123. Leelapornpisid, P., R. R. Wickett, S. Chansakaow, and N. Wongwattananukul. 2015. "Potential of native Thai aromatic plant extracts in antiwrinkle body creams." *Journal of Cosmetic Science* 66 (4): 219–31.

124. Valera, Marcia Carneiro, Lilian Eiko Maekawa, Luciane Dias de Oliveira, Antonio Olavo Cardoso Jorge, Érika Shygei, and Cláudio Antonio Talge Carvalho. 2013. "In vitro antimicrobial activity of auxiliary chemical substances and natural extracts on Candida albicans and Enterococcus faecalis in root canals." *Journal of Applied Oral Science* 21 (2): 118–23.

125. Maekawa, Lilian Eiko, Marcia Carneiro Valera, Luciane Dias de Oliveira, Cláudio Antonio Talge Carvalho, Carlos Henrique Ribeiro Camargo, and Antonio Olavo Cardoso Jorge. 2013. "Effect of Zingiber officinale and propolis on microorganisms and endotoxins in root canals." *Journal of Applied Oral Science* 21 (1): 25–31.

126. Ibid.

ABOUT THE AUTHOR

SUSAN BRANSON earned an undergraduate degree in biology from St. Francis Xavier University, then a MSc in toxicology from the University of Ottawa. From there, she worked in research: in the field, in the lab, as a writer, and as an administrator. She took time off and stayed at home after her second child was born. In addition to being a stay-at-home mom, she also took violin lessons, photography courses, earned a diploma in writing, and ultimately became a holistic nutritionist. Susan is a member of CSNN's Alumni Association, Canada's leading holistic nutrition school.

ABOUT FAMILIUS

VISIT OUR WEBSITE: WWW.FAMILIUS.COM

JOIN OUR FAMILY

There are lots of ways to connect with us! Subscribe to our newsletters at www.familius.com to receive uplifting daily inspiration, essays from our Pater Familius, a free ebook every month, and the first word on special discounts and Familius news.

GET BULK DISCOUNTS

If you feel a few friends and family might benefit from what you've read, let us know and we'll be happy to provide you with quantity discounts. Simply email us at orders@familius.com.

CONNECT

Facebook: www.facebook.com/paterfamilius
Twitter: @familiustalk, @paterfamilius1
Pinterest: www.pinterest.com/familius
Instagram: @familiustalk

FAMILIUS

> THE MOST IMPORTANT WORK YOU
> EVER DO WILL BE WITHIN THE
> WALLS OF YOUR OWN HOME.

CPSIA information can be obtained
at www.ICGtesting.com
Printed in the USA
FSOW02n0247060517
33833FS